The Age of Movement

Time Keeps On Moving and Why You Should Too

Dr. Beau Beard, DC, MS

E3 Publishing

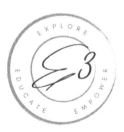

A huge thank you to my wife, Sloan, for always being my biggest fan. Maddyx, with my work I hope to make a positive impact on the world in order to leave it just a bit better for you.

Origin Story

I can still remember a light frost on the ground and the cold, damp ground against my back as I watched my leg twitch as it lay twisted and broken off to the side of my body. The year was 1993 and I was 9 years old. That morning I was playing pick-up football before school when a friend (yes, we are still friends) tackled me from behind, which caused a freak spiral fracture of my left femur. I was in the hospital for almost two weeks total, and on the fourth day a pediatric orthopedic surgeon was flown from Chicago to my small town hospital.

On that day, I was given two options. I could wear a cast that ran the entire length of my left leg, across my pelvis, and halfway down my right leg for 6-8 months, or inserting a titanium rod into the marrow cavity of my femur, then securing it with four screws.

Surprisingly enough, my parents let me choose which procedure I wanted. There had been many changes in my household in the past year, divorce, new parents and siblings, and the beginnings of far more autonomy than I ever knew I could handle. I believe that this scenario allowed my parents to feel comfortable with me choosing my fate. Whether it was the thought of wearing an uncomfortable and embarrassing cast for months on end or if my vast 9-year-old orthopedic knowledge sold me on the intramedullary rod, either way, I opted for the surgery. At the time I was only the ninth child to receive this surgery, and the original plan was to leave the rod in for 6 to 8 months and then remove it in a final surgery.

I spent another eight days in the hospital after the surgery. During that time, the only sliver of physical therapy that I received consisted of walking up three stairs using a railing, crossing a platform, and then walking back down three stairs. My physical therapists then coached me on using crutches properly, and then sent me on my way. I can only assume that my physicians thought that the resiliency of a 9-year-old body would trump any attempts at traditional physical therapy. Knowing what I know now, this was a misguided judgement that would determine a path, for better or worse, for the rest of my life.

My medical team laid out a few more precautions before I could head home. The first was never to play contact sports again. While highly unlikely, a second fracture of my femur could lead to amputation if the titanium rod became fractured or twisted. The thought of this terrified my mother. The second warning was that I should prepare to walk with a bit of a limp for the rest of my life. As if that was not enough, the doctors told me I would likely never run again.

So, that is what I was sent home with, a titanium rod, two crutches, the fear of God instilled in me of a possible future amputation, and the likelihood that I would never feel the wind against my face in a full out sprint. The next few weeks I was pampered and catered to by my parents and relatives. I openly welcomed the gifts, especially the food. Over the next month or so, I gained 15 pounds, 14 of which I am sure 90% could be contributed to Little Debbie snack cake consumption. At 9-years-old I had already become the modern-day picture of poor health, overweight, sedentary, and dealing with musculoskeletal pain and dysfunction. Thank God that I began to see the first glimpses of grit appear in my DNA at this pivotal point in my life.

My orthopedist recommended that I remain on crutches for six months. I was off them in half that time. After five months, I attempted to run with my friends, even though it looked more like a limping, hop-a-long type gait. At my six-month check-up, I was told that my bone was healing at an incredibly rapid pace. Knowing what I know now about physiology, loading of bone injuries early and often results in improved healing. While it seems like this should have been good news, it meant that my orthopedist wanted to leave the titanium rod in my leg. He explained that a second surgery would be far more traumatic than the first, and he assured me that doing so would not have any long-term ramifications.

Fast forward to my freshman year of high school. I had just finished my first football game. I had won the battle to play contact sports again. As we were reviewing the film of the game, my coach yelled out, "Beard, why in the hell are you limping? Are you hurt?". The thing was, I did not realize I was limping. The lack of physical therapy, possibly my impatience with crutches, and my obstinate and crude return to running had led to what I know now, is termed 'unconscious dysfunction.' Basically, I was completely unaware that I had developed a limp.

The next day at practice, now acutely aware of the hitch in my giddy-up as the unconscious dysfunction of my gait morphed into conscious dysfunction. The harder I tried to fix the issue, the more frustrated I grew. Finally, call it what you will, divine intervention, fate, or just dumb luck, but in 1999 a chiropractor and her husband that had been U.S. Judo National team had moved to my small town of Canton, IL. Dr. Kim and her husband, Reuben, came to our school to advertise their speed and agility camps, and I will never forget when Reuben did a backflip kick and hit the net on the basketball hoop. I was sold.

I signed up for the next camp that Dr. Kim and Reuben held. It was humbling to attend the speed camp with all of the other top athletes in my high school, and I found many of the exercises difficult and others that I could not do at all. By this point, my athleticism was developing, but my left leg was undeniably taking a toll on my ability to create speed and power. Another 'twist' of fate came in the form of a sprained ankle while playing basketball. My mother wanted me to see an orthopedist, but I had other plans.

The very next day, I was at Dr. Kim's office. While she immediately went to work on my ankle injury, she also pointed out some other things that I could work on to improve my overall movement and athletic prowess. Dr. Kim was far ahead of the field of chiropractic and physical therapy when it came to incorporating a gym, functional movement, and athletic training into a person's overall treatment and performance plan.

My ankle quickly bounced back, and I also noticed that the exercises Dr. Kim had me perform were translating over to the field of play. I was ecstatic to see appreciable change with the issue that had plagued me for so long, and I was now moving from conscious dysfunction to improved function. The true gold of my time with Dr. Kim was not found in obtaining unconscious function, but instead, it was the evolving clarity of my future career path. My struggles now carried more meaning, as I saw a way to ensure that a future me would have any and every opportunity not to lose the very thing that is so intimately intertwined with human life. Movement.

I am among the fortunate few led by early life experiences to prioritize movement, exercise, and health at a very young age. I eventually went to chiropractic school, and I have been in practice for almost a decade. Over the last twenty years, I have put my health first, but I have also been intrigued with pushing my body and mind beyond the generally accepted limits of our modern times. Doing so to provide personal proof that what I thought was once lost is still intact.

My goal for this book is to illustrate the vital role that movement plays in our lives as humans. Our relationship with our bodies has become disconnected and convoluted over the last few decades, and the only way to correct course is to increase our awareness. We must shift from a reactive health management model to a proactive optimization of our entire body, mind, and spirit.

Part I

State of the Human

1

Nature of the Beast

"Homo sapiens does its best to forget the fact, but it is an animal."
- Yuval Noah Harari

For most of modern human history, the idea of human movement has largely been taken for granted. It tends only to be those affected by movement impairment or loss who become keenly aware of just how vitally important movement is. The majority of us go about our lives walking, running, and playing with no need to examine our movement until it is affected by pain or dysfunction. We now find ourselves at an inflection point, and our relationship with movement has taken an unprecedented turn for the worst. Our kinesthetic aptitude has been a consistent and vital imperative for millenia, is now mutating into the most significant detriment to human health. To fully understand this emerging paradigm, we will first have to take a bit of a detour.

Steve Jobs famously stated that, "If you define the problem correctly, you almost have the solution". I think being healthy is best defined as the condition of being sound in body, mind, and spirit. This succinct definition gives us a holistic target to shoot for, but I think Moshé Feldenkrais gives us the most inspiring definition of all. "A healthy person is one who live fully his unavowed dreams".

The antithesis of good health is disease, and it comes as no surprise that humans, particularly Westernized humans, are more unhealthy than ever. While advances in medicine have lowered infant mortality and lengthened life expectancy, medicine has not provided humans with a defined path to health. Exactly how we got ourselves into this scenario and how we dig ourselves out of these unhealthy bodies and early graves is a complex and multifactorial endeavor. Even in the face of many impending global issues, it is hard to imagine a more important question than how to correct course on human health. Yet, we seem to continue to stray further away from a solution rather than move towards one.

Some of the more significant concerns at hand are obesity, chronic disease, substance abuse, and mental health issues. And there is a correlation. Daniel Lieberman, author of *The Story of the Human Body,* calls this condition 'mismatch diseases.' The mismatch hypothesis of environmental medicine attempts to answer why so many people are getting sick from previously rare illnesses, and the primary connection between the environments humans initially adapted to and our now maladaptive behavior, based on our current and wildly different setting. In essence, the very adaptations that helped bring us to our current state: the ability to store calories as fat, proficiency at creating and using tools, and our remarkable and unique consciousness, are all now being weaponized against us.

Simply put, humans have become ill-suited for their environment. The irony here is that humans have entirely created the current environment. For better or worse, we have made our bed, and now we have to lie in it. We have become the creators, curators, and protectors of an environment led by a societal devotion to growth and profit at the expense of health and vitality.

But at what cost?

To understand precisely what is happening to Homo sapiens, it may help to look at a strange adaptation occurring in an entirely different species, Bufo marinus or the Australian cane toad. The cane toad is a feral species native to South and Middle America introduced to Australia in 1935 by the Bureau of Sugar Experiment, to help control beetle populations. Since that time, the original 100 toads ballooned to more than 200 million. In a country known for its invasive species, the cane toad has become one of the greatest. During the cane toads precipitous procreation a peculiar adaptation took place.

The toads were not only increasing in number, but they also expanded the range they traveled. They evolved longer legs, greater endurance, and a tendency to move faster and further. However, while these adaptations provided the benefit of covering more territory to reproduce and establish a broader habitat, a trade-off occurred. These ultramarathoning toads now have shorter life spans and more spinal injuries due to their lengthened limbs. So why did these toads trade the ability to move faster and farther for shorter, more painful lives? Researchers at the University of Sydney's Richard Shine Lab determined that the process of "spatial sorting" was the culprit. Spatial sorting is analogous to survival of the fittest, with the ability to occupy space or territory being the determining factor of genetic success. Whereas, in a typical evolution model, the amount of time a species can keep its lineage alive is the primary factor. In this case spatial sorting led to a genetic surge of toads with these

Christoper Columbus-esque traits leading the forefront of the genetic battle for supremacy.

The exact reasons for the prioritization of spatial sorting over health and longevity are still not completely understood. Theories point to the fact that 'spatiotemporal fitness' or that organisms prioritize temporal fitness (longevity) and the ability to spread out and claim new territory over their own health. Sound familiar? I think we can all agree that if we had to give it up to humans in one arena, it would be that we have divided and conquered quite successfully. With 7.8 billion people covering almost every habitable space on the face of the Earth, and perhaps outer space, if we believe Elon Musk, we fall right in line with the concept of spatial sorting. Ever-expanding, but in a strange twist of fate, slowly killing ourselves and our environment in the process.

One of the cornerstones of human ability to successfully dominate an entire planet has been, and continues to be, our ability to develop and wield technology. Technology allows us to improve efficiency while decreasing manual labor demands. Watching how chimpanzees utilize the branch of a tree to fish termites out of a mound gives us an idea of just how far we have come, or perhaps how far we have fallen.

We have built a culture largely reliant on and addicted to technology that has made everything from obtaining food, working, and dating so devoid of physical connection or challenge that it is no wonder that this chasm of mismatch is occurring. Even though this technological trade-off has given humans the ability to travel the world, knock on the door of the cosmos, cure diseases that were once thought incurable, and connect almost every human across the face of the Earth, the price is steep. As humans alter the micro, meso, and macro environments of Earth to extents we didn't think possible, it seems that from the outside looking in, our world is no longer suitable for biological life. Elevated global temperatures, rising sea levels, and mass species extinction all point to a less human-friendly 'Blue Marble'. What if the reality is the fact that humans are now, far more ill-suited for life on Earth?

"In the end, it's not the years in your life that count. It's the life in your years".

You have probably heard this quote at some point, and no, it was not honest Abe, but instead Edward J. Stieglitz, M.D. While life expectancy in the West has continued to increase, with the current expectancy at 78.4 years, these added years are more typically filled with more disease and disability. Part of the reality of living longer is naturally facing more health issues due to "normal signs of aging," mainly attributed to cellular disorganization and dysfunction. As far as modern science can tell, this ultimately leads to our final sleep or senescence. However, the disease and disability that we are seeing occur is not happening in our golden years. Instead, we see major health issues occurring at much younger ages–propping up these morbidities with a healthcare system that is great at keeping the living from dying, but not as well suited at keeping the living healthy.

So, what exactly are the issues that are more commonly occurring at earlier ages?

According to The Centers for Disease Control and Prevention (interestingly, prevention wasn't added until 1992), the leading causes of death in the U.S. are heart disease and cancer, with accidents, respiratory disease, and stroke not far behind. Not surprisingly, the leading causes of these disorders are tobacco use, poor nutrition, excessive alcohol intake, and a *lack of physical activity.* It seems like an easy fix, as a species, we must stop smoking, drink less alcohol and replace it with water, eat a diet full of clean proteins, and move more. If so, then we could cause a dramatic decrease in morbidity and mortality rates. With such a simple solution, why hasn't more positive change occurred?

Why did congressionally supported anti-tobacco campaigns (1967) not snuff out smoking completely?

Why did federally mandated alcohol prohibition only last for 13 years (1920-1933)?

Why have the federal nutritional guidelines (first released in 1943) changed so much, and often supported advice in the face of competing evidence?

Why did Lyndon B. Johnson's Presidential Fitness Test (1966) not get us all moving more?

To understand the current health crisis, we need to explore further the underpinnings of major diseases and mortality causes and, as with most things, the best way to do that is to follow the money.

2
Why Movement

"Ignorance is the root cause of all difficulties."
- Plato

How can the nation with the most resources to treat medical issues lead the developed word in morbidity and mortality. How is that possible? Great strides have been made via the use of vaccines, antibiotics, and life-saving surgeries, but for the most part, the standard allopathic model is based on symptom relief and the maintenance of disease states. This is a great model for profit, but not so much for improving human health.

The irony here is that this is essentially how the U.S. medical system has been operating for the past century or so. If we take the top 10 killers in the U.S. annually (CDC, 2018) and combine the numbers of people affected, we get a total of more than 2 million people affected with approximately 1.5 trillion dollars spent on treatment. When comparing these totals to what we will call the 'Big 3' of declining health in the West, obesity, mental illness, and musculoskeletal disorders, sphincter tightening, and hyperventilation may ensue.

The total number of Americans dealing with obesity, mental health issues, or musculoskeletal disorders comes in at a whopping 236 million! With an aggregate annual price tag for care just north of $3.5 trillion. Essentially, 70% of the U.S. population is affected by the 'Big 3' and we spend 15% of the U.S. GDP (Gross Domestic Product) to prop up this broken medical system. Only 5% is spent on the top 10 causes of death combined. While this skewed focus leads to a failing system for millions of Americans; many of the issues that have been cornerstones of the U.S. health crisis are now starting to be seen globally.

Obesity is a perfect example of a mismatch disease. Advanced cognitive abilities, tool-wielding, and fantastic endurance led to success for hunter-gatherers for thousands of years. A key component of our nomadic endurance was the ability to store calories as fat to fuel us when food was scarce. Early hominids walked an average of ten kilometers per day, often in a fasted state. Such low-level aerobic movement allowed them to utilize fat stores to power their rather large brains and frail bodies. Ironically, our ability to store fat is no longer necessary in a world dominated by labor-saving technology and a dramatic reduction in human movement.

Global obesity numbers have tripled to 650 million, with a total of 1.9 billion people classified as overweight. In most countries, obesity now kills more people than starvation. There are so many layers to the global obesity epidemic. Farming practices create nutrient-devoid food while at the same time destroying the soil from which our food grows. A for-profit food industry hijacks our taste buds and neurochemistry to keep us eating food that takes us further away from optimal health. It is impossible to determine the exact cause of global human fattening, and it is hard to hit an undefined target when trying to correct course on such vital issues.

Mental health is an even more ominous threat to global health than obesity, with the worldwide affected rate coming in at just shy of one billion. One of the most troubling concerns with mental health disorders is the strong correlation to self-harm and suicide. According to a meta-analysis from the Journal of Affective Disorders in 2019, there is an eight-fold increased risk of suicide by those affected by mental illness. Suicide ranks as one of the top ten causes of death in the U.S. and the fourth leading cause of death in 15-19-year-olds worldwide. Again, the assumptions about what is driving the massive uptick in mental illness are numerous. Impending climate change and more social isolation in the face of more social media "connection" than ever, surely warrant some anxiety. Or does the issue go deeper than general social unrest?

Of the 'Big 3', musculoskeletal disorders are the absolute whopper of them all. With 1.71 billion people affected and the leading cause of disability worldwide, this is worth unraveling. What is a musculoskeletal (MSK) disorder? Generally speaking, MSK disorders are characterized by pain and limitation in mobility, dexterity, or overall level of function. MSK disorders are often divided into two subgroups: acute and chronic issues. Examples of acute disorders include things like sprains, strains, and fractures. Even in the face of expanding medical research and technology, acute injuries are still increasing across the globe.

Chronic conditions consist primarily of pain and functional adaptation or dysfunction that classically persists for more than six months. Of all the chronic MSK issues, low back pain ranks number one with over 568 million people affected worldwide, and is the leading cause of disability among all MSK disorders. It seems implausible to think that we live in a time where pain and mobility issues are perhaps the most significant problems we face as a species. Staring down climate change, war, human trafficking, pandemics fill in the blank for your modern-day woe, and it seems like your back pain should be the least of your worries. It does not take a medical professional to see the correlations between human movement and mental health, obesity, and the possible reduction of mismatch diseases. In 2017, the World Health Organization recognized just how dismal the outlook for MSK disorders had become and launched the Rehabilitation 2030 initiative. The goal is to increase global access to evidence-based rehabilitative services and resources on a large scale by the year 2030.

While the WHO's initiative is fantastic, it still reflects the reactive nature of the current medical model. Instead of increasing the resources for rehabilitation, what if we reduced the need for rehabilitation in the first place? The word rehabilitation comes from the Latin prefix *re-*, meaning "again", and *habitare*, meaning "make fit". To make fit again. Doesn't it seem more logical to never lose our fitness in the first place? To make the practice of *habitare* a lifelong habit.

In his book *The Tipping Point,* Malcolm Gladwell defined a "tipping point" as "the critical point in a situation, process, or system beyond which a significant and often unstoppable effect or change takes place". This may be our tipping point when it comes to the health and survival of current and future generations. Rather than continuing to react to issues like obesity and mental illness, why not try to understand their root causes and prevent their occurrence in the first place?

While movement and exercise are not a panacea for human health, they are vital to not only our survival but our ability to thrive. In a 7-year prospective cohort study from BioMed Central Medicine with over 150,000 participants, the data showed that cardiorespiratory fitness and muscle strength independently contribute to a lowered risk of mental health disease. We all inherently know that exercise makes you feel better, running, lifting, and swimming our way to saner and less stressed states of being. A study out of the University of Colorado demonstrated that exercise was a better tool for losing, and more importantly, keeping weight off. The research from this study determined that exercise acts as an energy regulation factor, and not just a caloric burn effect. Once people began to exercise, they tended to keep moving more often.

Motion is lotion, and rest is rust.

This is where a clear delineation needs to occur between the concepts of movement and exercise. Movement is using your body to operate within your environment to achieve tasks and maintain survival successfully. For eons, hominids have crawled, walked, climbed, carried, and ran to hunt, eat, evade, and play. It was not until the modern era that exercise became part of everyday human life. From the Latin root *exercitium* meaning training or play, we can discern that exercise was initially utilized to hone skills that furthered survival. While survival and health are linked, they are not one and the same.

An ancient Greek warrior working on swordsmanship, a Native American shooting a bow from horseback, or a Neanderthal practicing their atlatl marksmanship before a hunt, are all examples of training that was necessary to stay alive. Training bleeds into practice, and practice morphs into sport. Examples of sport are seen throughout human history, from Greeks wrestling at the Olympics, Iroquois playing stickball, to Persians playing polo. It seems that sport has always been part of modern human life. Sport allows humans to put those same survival skills to the test on a contrived field of battle where the consequences are usually far less severe.

Sport has transformed from the days of testing our skills against fellow men to assure proficiency in other, often more meaningful tasks, a playground with a guided path to professionalism. Pressurization of the your sports model has come mainly in the form of increased competition for the elusive D1 athletic scholarship. The financial gain and social recognition of achieving a full or even partial athletic scholarship is just one more form of 'keeping up with the Joneses.

Unfortunately, it is common to put the cart before the horse and start training for sport before achieving movement competency. This mismanagement of priorities comes with a cost. It is this mindset that is partially responsible for the fivefold increase in youth sports injuries since 2010. Physical therapist and author Gray Cook extols this piece of advice in his book titled *Movement*, "first move well, then move often". Particularly in America, we have flipped this equation on its head regarding athletics and sport, and even more so in the desperate attempt to regain fitness and shed some pounds later in life.

Movement is the antecedent to exercise and sport, and approximately 70% of all human movement follows a predestined path, from birth to our first steps. This process of biological maturation, or ontogenesis, is married to our genetically encoded movement blueprint. Unlike many other mammals in the animal kingdom, humans do not exit the womb with a fully formed movement vocabulary. Instead, it takes years to develop and master the basic movements that will be with us for the rest of our lives. These movement engrams, or cognitive patterns, may be crucial to our continued health and survival throughout lifetime.

Researchers from the University of Missouri have found evidence that regular exercise allows our genome to be expressed more thoroughly and efficiently throughout a lifetime. It is almost as if movement and exercise are the keys that unlock our true humanness. Tapping into long-established movement requisites that have evolved over hundreds of thousands of years keeps the trillions of cells in our bodies working and communicating as efficiently as possible. Simple things like walking, lifting something heavy a few times a week, and elevating your heart rate every now and again have been shown to stave off everything from type II diabetes to dementia.

It is worth noting that exercise and movement are only part of a holistic approach to human health. In fact, a clinical review of over 150 studies with over 300,000 participants out of Brigham Young University showed that friendship, especially later in life, was the most critical factor when it came to improved health and mortality rates. The same study showed that having fewer friends had a more negative effect on health than being obese or not exercising. For simplicity's sake, we can categorize human health into seven main facets or what I refer to as the pillars of health: movement, spirit, nutrition, sleep, purpose, relationships, and the mind. This expansion on the standard definition of human health of body, spirit, and mind allows us to become more precise when determining and discussing what comprises optimal health.

In the following pages, I have two goals. I first want to present a guide on human movement from birth to death. Think of this as the Human Movement Manual. Second, I will show how movement is not just a part of, but a critical component to all seven pillars of human health and quite possibly a rather large piece of the puzzle when it comes to remedying our current health crisis. To do so, we will have to journey back in time a bit to accomplish both, only about 3.5 billion years ago.

3
The First Movement

"And the earth was without form, and void; and darkness was upon the face of the deep. And the Spirit of God moved upon the face of the waters."
- Genesis 1:2

The proverbial calendar of life for planet Earth has been peeled back at regular intervals over the last few decades, as scientists keep discovering exactly how far back life extends. It has long been thought that life on Earth has existed for approximately 3.5-3.7 billion years. During these earliest moments of life, microbes flourish in a world elementally devoid of oxygen and high in methane. According to research from the National Academies of Science, around 2.5 billion years ago, signs of the earliest cyanobacteria start to emerge, which were the Earth's first photo-synthesizers. These photon-converting microbes catalyze a massive environmental shift that will change the world forever. Cyanobacteria (which still exist today in blue-green algae) release oxygen as a byproduct, which is responsible for most known life on Earth today.

This cosmic breath of fresh air, or the "Great Oxidation Event," sets the stage for the Earth's first biological movements. Like many great firsts, the first primitive movers did not do so in isolation. Instead, it took cooperation among many single-cell organisms. West African rock formations show fossilized burrows where eukaryotes cooperated to form slug-like multicellular organisms. With a bit of teamwork and oxygen to fuel the movement fire, these primordial movers were off and running or at least slimily crawling.

This eukaryotic team-up was more along the lines of one organism ingesting the other. The first multicellular organisms work together through endosymbiosis, which become the precursory model for future internal organs. A few of these internal organs or organelles become crucial to the first evolutionary steps towards complex life on Earth. DNA storage became possible by forming the cell nucleus, allowing for the packaging of easily transferable information through the most rudimentary forms of sexual reproduction.

The other breakthrough organ was mitochondria. You probably remember learning in grade school that the mitochondria are the 'powerhouse' of the cell. Along with the crucial production of adenosine triphosphate or ATP, the mitochondria are critical signaling agents to other cells that relay information about diseases and eventual cellular death. With photosynthesizing cells that were capable of procreating and passing along their genetic material to future generations, the need for what Walter Rosen of the National Research Council first termed 'biodiversity' now become apparent.

As complexity and diversity within these prehistoric organisms grows, divisions become apparent between plants, fungi, and animals. While this occurred approximately 900 million years ago, I will take chronological liberties here and skip ahead 200 million years, where we begin to see the earliest ancestors of modern-day jellyfish form. These jellies or cnidarians are the first animals that need to remain in constant motion to acquire oxygen and food. Thus, movement has officially become synonymous with life.

Skipping ahead, we now find ourselves 570 million years ago, and this is where we see a group of animals called *Ambulacraria* emerge. These invertebrates are the earliest forms of starfish, and they were given their name due to the feet or podia contained within their ambulacral groove. The starfish's archaic but practical form of ambulation has not changed in over half a billion years–the perfect example of highly effective yet simplistic design by mother nature.

As divisions between invertebrates and vertebrates begin to emerge, the earliest vertebrate evolves from a jawless fish, similar to the modern-day hagfish. For the next 70 million years or so, the ocean seems to be the party scene. Then, approximately 500 million years ago, a cousin of insects and cephalopods is thought to emerge from the sea to be the first animal to ever crawl on dry land. An explosion of life is about to change the face of our great planet, but it is not animals that take the early lead in this race for life.

Thought to be yet another vital step in the evolutionary process to sustain complex life, around 465 million years ago, plants colonize almost every corner of the Earth. At this point, plant life allows for the oxygen-carbon dioxide cycle to catalyze even more oxygen production within the atmosphere. Thus, it is worth noting that our modern-day success as a species is primarily owed to our ability to utilize oxygen.

Shortly after plants spread across the planet, we see an explosion of insect life, and if the theory holds, the earliest forms of bony fish such as *Tiktaalik* emerged on land. *Tiktaalik* was a mix between fish and tetrapod, with vestigial limbs and the ability to breathe via both gills and lungs. Once tetrapods emerged onto dry land, it was game over. Three hundred eighty-five million years ago, the first four-legged animals began to dominate the scene and have ever since. Since crawling on dry land has been a movement staple of animals for a few hundred million years, maybe it is unwise to rush our babies through this ancient and fundamental stage of movement? More on that topic to come later.

During this same period, evidence of the first trees emerges, and yet another major environmental oxygen contributor has arrived. Although the evolutionary timelines appear using various species to dictate when and what was occurring, it seems that life emerging on land is immediately followed by dinosaurs roaming the land. Examining the fossil record reveals that this is not quite the case.

It takes approximately another 70 million years to see the earliest dinosaurs emerge alongside other early forms of reptiles and amphibians. Moving forward in time to 200 million years ago, we see the fourth mass extinction occur on Earth. Yes, up to this point, there had been three other mass extinction events, with the third being the most significant on record. The Permian extinction wipes out 96% of species on Earth, which eventually sets the stage for the domination of dinosaurs. Dinosaurs will rule the Earth for the next 140 million years or so, but alongside them, early mammals develop warm-bloodedness, the first flowering plants show up, and early forms of birds emerge. More critical to Homo sapiens eventual dominance is the appearance of early mammals such as rodents and hares, of which some species eventually survive the fifth mass extinction.

Sixty-five million years ago, the Cretaceous-Paleogene extinction wipes out approximately 75% of all species on Earth, thus paving the way for the era of mammal dominance. It is worth noting that modern-day arthropods (insects, crustaceans, and arachnids) currently outnumber mammals by a ratio of 312 to 1 and plant life by 17 to 1. It's their world, and we just live in it. Only 2 million years later, we see a split occur between mammals. This division leaves us with two subsets of primates; the wet-nosed and the dry-nosed variety. The wet-nosed primates evolve into modern species of lemurs and aye-ayes, while the dry-nosed type develop into monkeys, apes, and eventually humans.

Over the next 40 million years, many branches of the evolutionary tree sprout, giving shape to both modern-day land and sea animals. Finally, around 6 million years ago, we see a defining split amongst primates that leads to eventual human life. At this point, Sahelanthropus tchadensis or some other early hominid split from chimpanzees and bonobos to then begin the bipedal journey toward Homo erectus. However, it would take more than 5 million years for the earliest traces of early humans to show up in the fossil record.

Somewhere on the African savanna, early Homo sapiens emerged from a lineage of other hominids such as Neanderthal and Denisovans. Since that time, we have become the preeminent force of the planet. While it took hundreds of millions of years to swim, slither, crawl, and eventually walk our way into the evolutionary timeline, humans are still very young in the grand scheme of things. Our evolutionary immaturity may be one of the critical links to the current plight we find ourselves in as a species today.

At present we are living in the Holocene epoch, but many researchers and scientists have long debated that we may be actually inhabiting the Anthropocene, or the "the human epoch". While still not formally accepted by many scientists as a legitimate epoch, many believe that this human era began at one of a few jumping-off points, such as the agricultural revolution almost 15,000 years ago or the Industrial Revolution of the 1800s. However, many researchers think that the detonation of the first atomic bomb in 1945 serves as the best timestamp for the beginning of the Anthropocene. Regardless of the date of origin, it is hard to deny that humans dominate this current era, and the global transformation we have brought about may sadly tip the scales toward yet another mass extinction.

In only the last few centuries, humans have reshaped the environment and, therefore, our lives so that it almost seems we are not welcome in the very home we built. Harvard professor and the father of sociobiology, E.O. Wilson, said it best, "The real problem of humanity is the following: we have Paleolithic emotions, medieval institutions, and god-like technology." We are evolutionary kindergarteners, finger-painting with environmental weapons of mass destruction.

"Complaining about a problem without posing a solution is called whining" is an oft-quoted line by Teddy Roosevelt. So, to not just stand in the corner and play my tiny violin, I suppose it is time to propose a solution. What an audacious task to pose a solution to global health issues, with the thought that correcting the course on human health may have a ripple effect on some of the other great maladies of our time. I aim to do this, and at the heart of this proposed solution is human movement.

The mathematical concept of an elegant solution is one that achieves the maximally satisfactory outcome with minimal effort. While I would like to lull you into the idea of providing an elegant solution to our current health dilemma, I believe this way of thinking is what brought us to this tipping point in the first place. Just as humans would rather store calories and save energy, mind you by evolutionary design, by developing technology, systems, and artificial intelligence to accomplish just that. We may have to deny the Darwinian urges that turn us into obese, techno-crazed zombies and instead reacquaint ourselves with our bodies. Seek discomfort in the face of living in a world where comfort is the status quo. Explore the connections occurring inside ourselves, among others, and within our environment. Then we may begin to fully understand and utilize the body gifted to us.

To obtain knowledge and not use it is idiocy; to act upon acquired knowledge is wisdom. So before we can do or, in this case, move, we must first learn. Part II of this book is a guide, the Human Movement Manual. This guide will take you from the womb to death, with detailed specifications on what comprises normal movement at each stage of life, why each step is necessary, and a few tips along the way on how to maintain, regain, and maximize your movement and health.

Part II

Human Movement Guide

1

In Utero

"There are many events in the womb of time which will be delivered."
-William Shakespeare

The Lummi Nation, also known as the Lhaq'temish or 'People of the Sea,' is a Native American tribe that calls Washington state home. The Lummi believe that the stories, beliefs, and culture that an expectant mother is exposed to somehow program these things into the DNA of a baby within the womb. This process helps young Lummi carry on the cultural traditions by weaving them into their very being via cellular programming.

The Lummi have a deep-seated belief in the process of genetic imprinting through traditions and stories. As it often occurs throughout human history, rituals and customs often precede the science that seemingly legitimizes them. Nevertheless, science and data have begun to emerge looking at the effects that things like music, emotions, trauma, and exercise have on a human in utero, as an infant, and later into childhood. This type of passing of the genetic torch is called intergenerational epigenetic inheritance.

The human story has always started with movement, and as a species, we have a particular penchant for one type of movement in particular (wink, wink). Some theorists even believe that sex may have been the most potent driver behind verbal communication, art, and higher-order cognitive processing. Imagine the beginning of a triathlon, thousands of swimmers elbowing, kicking, and punching their way over the top of one another through the water to be the first onshore. This image encapsulates the movement of millions of viable sperm carrying a father's genetic expression–traveling the approximate 18 centimeters to make their way through the cervix with one lucky swimmer finally fertilizing the expectant egg. This journey is technically the first human movement, the cellular dash for genetic legacy.

Once fertilization occurs, even as movement abounds with rapid cellular replication, this is our germination stage, or we can think of it as our first introduction to meditation. Although there is relatively little movement related to a young fetus up until about 18 weeks of gestation, this is when the movement spark ignites, only to be extinguished when we exit on the other side of life.

At this point in the womb, the fetal movement consists of kicks, punches, thumb sucking, rolling, and the notorious hiccups that can occur up to 30 times per hour. While hiccups in adulthood are a common annoyance, they are vital for developing the thoracic diaphragm while in utero. Many first-time mothers are quite surprised by the strange and powerful sensation that fetal hiccups produce. These small but powerful contractions of the thoracic diaphragm are crucial to developing this muscle which is the major player in our breathing function after birth. We will discuss the pivotal role of the diaphragm more in the upcoming chapters.

Each of these movements may seem random, but they all have their unique purpose. For instance, sucking the thumb and touching the lower face indicate healthy neurologic development and builds the sucking power needed for successful breastfeeding immediately after birth.

Kicks and punches coincide with the intrauterine growth cycle when bones and joints form. These karate-like movements apply stress to the neonate musculoskeletal system creating appropriate maturation. This adaptation is called Wolff's law and is the same principle applied throughout life to develop strong and resilient bones in response to stressors such as lifting weights or running.

While all of these intrauterine martial arts and breath-work are taking place, we hope that mom gets her fair share of movement and exercise as well. Believe it or not, there was a time when pregnancy was almost treated as an illness; women were told to eliminate any vigorous activity and ordered to bed rest at the slightest sign of a problem in many cases. But times, they are a-changin'.

It is now common knowledge that those who exercise – including pregnant women – tend to have lower resting heart rates than those who do not. Lower resting heart rates can signify an efficient heart; higher resting heart rates have been linked to a greater risk of cardiovascular disease and stroke. In a 2010 study out of East Carolina University, researchers collected a group of 26 pregnant women who reported that they had been exercising three times a week for more than 30 minutes per session. When researchers brought the expectant mothers into the lab at 36 weeks, they found that the fetuses, too, had lower heart rates than those carried by the moms who were not regular exercisers.

Results like these may indicate that exercise during pregnancy can be incredibly beneficial for both mom and baby, a far cry from harming the fetus. And timing matters: exercise *during* pregnancy, instead of pre-

pregnancy fitness, seems to be doing something extra-special. In this most recent study, about half of the group had not exercised previously and still saw similar effects on their babies' hearts.

These heart benefits may last into a child's early life. For example, the same research found that month-old infants up to 6-year-old children showed higher heart rate variability and higher ejection fractions (which indicates hearts are pumping blood more efficiently) if they had exercised with their mothers in utero.

As previously mentioned, the effects of exercise and movement do not only affect the cardiovascular system. In another study, mothers in their first trimester were randomly assigned to either an exercise or a sedentary control group. The ten women in the exercise group cycled, walked, ran, or swam for three short sessions a week, pushing themselves hard enough to get slightly out of breath. The eight women in the sedentary group were told not to exercise. In the 8 to 12 days after the babies were born, the researchers measured their brain activity. They recorded electroencephalograms (EEG) while they played the sleeping babies a series of beeps interspersed with different sounds. Even though the babies were asleep, patterns in their brain activity showed how efficiently they could discriminate between old versus novel sounds. More developed brains find the task easier than less mature ones. To summarize, babies born from physically active mothers have a more mature cerebral activation, suggesting that their brains developed more rapidly.

Just as the Lummi people believe that unborn children have their stories and culture woven into their DNA, our movement story as humans may be written long before conception occurs. There has been evidence that if, and to what extent people and other animals move depends to some degree on family history and genetics. For example, past twin studies and genome-wide association studies suggest that about 50 percent of physical activity behavior in people may depend on genes. In addition to our base genetic code, we know that each human is endowed with 4-5 million SNP's or single nucleotide polymorphisms. These SNP's, in essence, allow genes to be turned 'on' or 'off.' These genetic variations are attributed to many variables, with the largest coming from our parents, grandparents, and even great grandparents. The idea that the lifestyle and environment that your predecessors were exposed to can have a trait-based trickle-down effect is known as intergenerational epigenetics.

In his book Biology of Belief, Bruce Lipton, Ph.D. states that, "Adaptive mutation implies purposefulness in biological evolution". These adaptive mutations are literally what made and continue to make us human. Our DNA is beckoning for us to move, before we were born, the echoes of our need to move were whispered to the cells of our ancestors. Just as the Lummi dance to their indigenous music and speak stories in their native tongue to pass on their culture. As humans, we must honor our ancestral DNA by moving and exercising to pass on our movement story, our human story.

2
0-6 Months

"Every child begins the world again."
- Henry David Thoreau

Homo sapiens may have evolved as the most complex creatures on the planet, but this complexity comes at a price. Humans are vulnerable and utterly dependent on their parent(s) at birth, especially in comparison with many of our mammalian cousins. Conjure the scene of a wildebeest birth on the Serengeti, or an elk calf in Yellowstone, even a litter of puppies at your local pet store; all of these offspring are born with about the same capacity for movement as their adult parents. Even our closest evolutionary cousins, chimpanzees and bonobos, are born with a modicum of motor control and independent movement.

We sacrifice early movement proficiency to lay an intricate and still somewhat misunderstood foundation for our central nervous system. We hone our vision, equilibrium, breathing, and postural-locomotion patterns during the first year of human life. These neurological developments are subcortical, meaning that they are very primitive functions that have been prevalent in humans and many mammalian ancestors for millennia. It has been postulated by Professor Pavel Kolar, the director of the rehabilitation department at the University Hospital Motol School of Medicine in Prague, that "the level and quality of the central nervous system(CNS) maturation corresponds with the level and quality of motor patterns". Therefore, by simply observing a newborn's movement patterns, it is postulated that one may be able to determine the health of a human's nervous system. The central nervous system does not reach full maturity until around the 5th to 6th year of life, but our external expression of our internal neurology persists for a lifetime. As neuroscientist Daniel Wolpert puts it, "We have a brain for one reason and one reason only – that is to produce adaptable and complex movements".

The first observed movement in almost every human on earth is that of our first breath. That first shrill cry that every parent nervously awaits, bringing with it a sigh of relief that labor is over and a seemingly healthy baby has made its world debut. The breath that precedes that first wail is the first of approximately 700 million breaths to be taken throughout the rest of a human's life. Breath is our first independent movement, and it sets the stage for all other movements to come.

Nuchal Cord

Let me reiterate, *almost* every human begins with a breath. Anywhere from 25-40% of babies are born with the umbilical cord wrapped around their neck or what is called a nuchal cord. I was one of those babies, which has driven many of my fascinations with breathing as it pertains to human function and health throughout a lifetime.

Shortly after birth, most babies are run through the Apgar Scoring system, which addresses Appearance Pulse Grimace Activity Respiration.

When looking at these five vital criteria, it becomes apparent just how crucial movement is to human health and well-being, with three of the five categories addressing some sort of movement.

The 'Activity' portion of testing addresses muscle tone and resistance to stress, 'Breathing' looks at the ease or difficulty of breathing, and 'Grimace' response is simply the response of the newborn to mild stimuli such as a skin prick or gentle pinch, with the expected result being a cough, sneeze or vigorous activity. This is the first of many primitive reflexes assessed and used to ascertain an infant's neurological and developmental status in the first few months of life. See the inserted chart for reference.

*Keep in mind that typical gestation = 40 weeks. **These are all taken from the TherapyEd prep book (pgs 116-117)

BIRTH	1 MO	2 MO	3 MO	4 MO	5 MO	6 MO	7 MO	8 MO	9 MO	10 MO	11 MO	12 MO	2 YRS	5 YRS	PERSISTS
Spinal Galant (32 wks – 2mo)															
Rooting (28 wks - 3mo)															
Suck-swallow (28 wks – 2-5mo)															
Traction (28 wks – 2-5mo)															
Palmar Grasp (37 wks – 4-6 mo)															
MORO (28 wks – 4-6mo)															
ATNR (37 wks – 4-6 mo)															
Tonic Labyrinthine (TLR) (37 wks – 6mo)															
Plantar grasp (28 wks – 9 mo)															
Head righting (birth-2mo – PERSISTS)															
			Landau (3-4mo – 12-24mo)												
				STNR (4-6mo – 8-12 mo)											
				Neck righting (NOB) (4-6 mo – 5 years)											
				Body on body righting (BOB) (4-6 mo – 5 years)											
				↓DOWNWARD protective extension (parachute) (4 mo – PERSISTS)											
					Prone tilting (5 mo – PERSISTS)										
						→FORWARD protective extension (6-9mo – PERSISTS)									
							←→SIDEWAYS protective extension (7mo – PERSISTS)								
							Supine/sitting tilting (7-8mo – PERSISTS)								
									←BACKWARD protective extension (9-10mo – PERSISTS)						
									Quadruped tilting (9-12mo – PERSISTS)						
												Stand tilting (12-21mo – PERSISTS)			

As with many things, the old becomes new again, and the practice of 'breast crawling' has made its way back into the popular culture spotlight. This interesting phenomenon takes place when the newborn is placed on the mother's abdomen and instinctively crawls up to her breast and usually latches on to the nipple for their very first feeding. It is postulated that it can aid in bonding, the expulsion of the placenta, lactation, and even a lowered risk of postpartum depression. This was a part of the birthing process for millenia, although this was first described in the literature by, Widström et al., 1987, "these findings suggest that an organized feeding behavior develops predictably during the first hours of life".

This type of predictable and instinctive movement is what is so incredibly interesting about the development of human movement. With no coaching and little outside influence besides environmental factors, 70% (Kolar et al., 2013) of babies will follow the same kinesiological development. It is simply awe-inspiring to think that the complexity of human movement is programmed right into our genetic code.

The first four weeks of life, or the neonatal stage, comprises 'general' movements. These non-specific movements are thought to be the external representations of central nervous system development. It is almost as if we can see the sparks fly as millions of synaptic connections and neuroplastic changes develop to build our movement vocabulary. A handful of movements characterize the neonatal stage, most of which are regulated by the aforementioned primitive reflexes. The following are a few examples of these reflexive movements that are typically seen in a developing neonate.

The cross-extension reflex can be elicited by flexing an infant's hip and knee while they are lying on their back. In a healthy baby, this will prompt the opposite leg to extend or straighten. Another primitive reflex present during this time is the Babkin reflex which can be produced by applying pressure into the newborn's palm with the expected reaction of mouth opening and head-turning toward the side of stimulus. These are just a few examples of subcortically regulated movements present during the first four weeks of life.

It should also be noted that the persistence of certain primitive reflexes beyond this stage can be just as indicative of pathology as a present reflex is of normal development. Other characteristics of this stage include optical fixation for only a few seconds and a predilection to which side the head turns. Neonates can turn their head volitionally, but when the head turns passively, the rest of the body will follow. This type of movement has been deemed 'holokinetic.'

It is essential to point out that developmental milestones vary in every baby, with a typical variance range of plus or minus six weeks. There is absolutely no benefit to hitting a developmental milestone early. Although it may happen, it does not mean that your child is destined to be a professional athlete. Encouraging children to sit, stand or walk early is more than likely detrimental to their development. So throw out your bouncy chairs and stop hanging your kids from their arms to walk like marionette puppets!

As the first month of life comes to a close, movement progress begins to quicken pace. In the 4-6 week stage, babies start to lift their heads against gravity, but this movement is still holokinetic in nature. When lying on their stomach at this stage, the infant can begin to support their body on their forearms, and when lying supine, they can start to lift their legs off the ground for short periods. The predilection position of the head fades, and the baby emerges into a typical posture deemed 'fencer's position.' Imagine a baby lying on its back; head turned toward one side with the same side arm reaching out as if thrusting a sword. In addition to these simple movements, some primitive reflexes disappear in a typically developing infant, such as stepping automation, Babkin, and heel reflex.

From two months to six months of age, a host of changes takes place. First, muscular co-activation, or equal activation of agonist and antagonist muscles, occurs, allowing for the first signs of upright posture. At three months of age, a baby can lift the trunk from the forearms and look up into cervical and thoracic extension. Muscular co-activation and uprighting are primarily possible due to creating adequate Intra Abdominal Pressure (IAP). IAP is pressure that is built in the abdomen as the thoracic diaphragm descends toward the pelvic floor, and the concomitant muscular resistance of the abdominal wall to this pumping action. IAP subsequently creates efficient and dynamic stability in the developing baby. With this newly found pressurization, babies continue to work on lifting the legs and pelvis further from the ground, developing the abdominal chains and allowing for more central stability.

Diastasis Recti

Diastasis rectus abdominis (DRA) is a separation between the left and right rectus abdominis or, more generally considered, a form of hernia. DRA is usually associated with postpartum women who have had excess stretching on the abdominal wall, particularly the tissue between the recti called the linea alba. DRA occurs in approximately 60% of women, but this can also occur in males with excess abdominal adiposity or other functional deficits leading to increased anterior abdominal wall loading. As this pertains to developmental kinesiology, technically, all babies use

42

the time from 3-8 months to shore up the abdominal wall, and disturbances during this developmental stage may contribute to future findings of DRA.

While diastasis recti may appear symptomless in most people, it is an important finding as it correlates to central stability strategy. As mentioned in chapter one, creating adequate intra-abdominal pressure is crucial to an effectively stabilize our bodies as we develop higher levels of coordination. In addition, DRA can contribute to excess compression on the lumbar spine, which may be correlated with future pain or injury. Regardless of the cause of DRA, there are many viable ways to work on this issue to limit future problems associated with it.

With more sagittal plane stability at hand, a baby can now move upper and lower extremities more efficiently, allowing for better interaction with external objects. At this period of time, babies will also be able to grip actively, specifically gaining the ability to grab outside of their midline. Seeking and grabbing toys or objects outside midline is crucial for the next major milestone of rolling.

Around the five-month mark (remember it could be sooner or later), babies will begin to be able to roll from supine to prone and prone to supine. Rolling from back to front, babies will start moving from an ipsilateral pattern, where both upper and lower extremities are moving in the same direction, to more contralateral or reciprocal patterns, where the upper and lower extremities move in opposite directions. In general, humans are built to move with asymmetrical contralateral patterns such as walking and running. We all know that before you can run, you have to walk, and before you walk, you have to crawl.

3
6-12 Months

"If you can't fly then run, if you can't run then walk, if you can't walk then crawl, but whatever you do you have to keep moving forward."
- Dr. Martin Luther King, Jr.

While this quote is inspirational, it seems to deem crawling as an inferior choice of movement. Well, that is just not the case.

Have you ever been around parents who beamed with pride as they happily boasted about the fact that their baby walked early, or better yet, skipped crawling all together! Well, folks, not only is this something not to be proud of, but it may be detrimental to your child's development. Hitting each developmental window on time is vital to proper physiologic and neurologic development. Each developmental stage has been coded into human DNA for thousands and thousands of years to allow our anatomy and neurology to develop appropriately.

Before a baby crawls, many movement milestones occur to set the stage for independent mobility. For example, at approximately the 5-6 month mark, a baby can achieve the yoga termed 'happy baby' position and arguably the best plank they will ever perform. At this stage, they can also roll from supine to prone. While babies' proportions do not match their adult counterparts, such as legs that are much shorter than adults in relation to their torso, it is easy to accomplish these tasks–attributed to the exceptionally unadulterated central stability developed in the early months of human life.

To add to the importance of not skipping developmental stages, it's worth noting how the popularized 'tummy time' plays into the eventual crawling phase as well as scapulothoracic (shoulder/shoulder blade) stability throughout a lifetime. If a baby does not spend enough time loading the scapulothoracic and glenohumeral joints in the 2-5 month range, a plethora of issues can surface. Proceeding into crawling without this crucial stability building time can result in altered movement patterns, decreased mobility/stability, as well as possible pain and injury as things like sports and activities of daily living are introduced. So while babies may not always enjoy lying face down on a play mat, it is vital!

Around the 6-7 month mark, babies will begin to crawl. Crawling is the foundation for the variety of contralateral-based movements that occur throughout our adult life, such as walking and running. Crawling calls upon all of the other pieces that have been put into place up to this point, such as adequate intra-abdominal pressure and upper and lower extremity coordination that has been grooved in the motor cortex and integrated with the cerebellum. It's interesting to note that in the world of rehabilitation, both for adults and children, when the ability to crawl is lost, it can be a sign of either significant neurologic issues or severe movement restriction due to disuse.

Crawling is one of the first vital stages of movement development necessary to properly form the two most mobile joints of the body, the hip, and the shoulder. In addition to developing these ball and socket joints, sesamoid bones such as the patella or kneecap, which derives its moniker from sesame seed, begin to develop during this phase of life. You have other sesamoid bones in your body, and just with any other bone, Wolff's law determines that when a bone is stressed, it responds to the demand by creating a solid and resilient trabecular and cortical structure. While the patella doesn't fully fuse until the age of 5-6, the transition from cartilage to bone begins during this crucial period.

These primal movements are vital for creating musculoskeletal and neurologic functions, and evidence shows that they may have ties to emotional development as well. Research out of the Harvard School of Medicine shows that the cerebellum participates in limbic-related functions. The cerebellum, Latin for 'little brain,' is the movement coordination center of the hindbrain. The limbic system, also known as the paleomammalian cortex, is an ancient set of brain structures that regulate emotions, behavior, long-term memory, and our sense of smell.

As babies begin to incorporate more of these contralateral or cross-crawl patterns into their movement repertoire, a need for more communication across hemispheres of both the cerebrum and cerebellum occurs. At this point in life cross patterning is powerful at this point in life for the development of emotions and behavior. Also, it can be utilized later in life to tap into these primal brain areas for anxiety relief. One of the more complex cross-crawl patterns humans develop is running, and the runner's high is an oft sought-after endorphin rush that can go toe-to-toe with some the most commonly prescribed anti-anxiety medication out there.

This newfound mobility creates a much bigger environmental pallet from which the baby can now interact. Therefore, the continual development of babies is mainly dependent on a safe, secure, and stimulating environment.

From 7-9 months of age, babies will explore various movements that will follow them like a shadow for the rest of their lives. For example, side sitting helps develop the external and internal rotators of the hip, which will be necessary for eventual upright posture and walking. We also start to see the first signs or verticalization as babies begin to sit upright without aid and then progress to pulling themselves into a tripod or half-kneeling position. These positions set the stage for independent use of both hands in an upright posture, another developmental leap for enhanced environmental interaction.

From months 8-10, babies will start crawling to a different vertical position, commonly referred to as 'bear' or a 'bear crawl.' This position allows for further independent isolation of each limb and greater stability demand across the entire kinematic chain. From bear position, babies will graduate to the modern-day version of movement wealth, the deep squat.

It's interesting to note cultural differences in movement, such as the deep squat, which is often referenced as the 'Asian' squat. In many Eastern cultures, this position is used during resting, socializing, and using the bathroom. However, in Western culture, we often see children as young as 8-years-old may start to lose their ability to adopt the flat-footed deep squat that seems oh-so-comfortable when observing our Eastern counterparts. Due to Western culture's use of things like elevated heeled shoes, seats that allow babies to verticalize before adequate stability development, and the seated postures we adopt throughout a large portion of our lives, it's almost as if American's undergo squat amnesia. So the adage of "if you don't use it, you lose it" definitely rings true in this case.

From the deep squat position, children begin to adopt a standing posture, often using a stabilizing aid such as a table, chair, or parent at first. Just as it was discussed with crawling earlier, aided walking by hanging children from their arms or the use of walkers is strongly discouraged. Putting a child into a developmental position that is too advanced for their developmental age can adversely affect their movement progress. We can consider that a ubiquitous movement mandate by now.

Once a baby can stand with the aid of a stabilizing feature, ambulation will start to take place in the frontal plane or side-to-side. With eventual movement occurring in the transverse or rotational plane as they begin to turn away from that stabilizing aid.

From here on out, the race is on.

4
1-2 Years

"A person does not grow from the ground like a vine or a tree, one is not part of a plot of land. Mankind has legs so it can wander."
- Roman Payne, The Wandresss

As the developmental stage name implies, toddlers are not gracefully strolling through their world. That by no means stops them from exploring every inch of their environment, finding every sharp corner, uncovered outlet, and any number of life-threatening predicaments to get themselves into. Walking is truly our first glimpse at independence, but hold back the tears, there is still a long journey ahead.

From approximately 11 to 15 months, toddlers are pretty clumsy and therefore must quickly master the art of falling. These sometimes painful early struggles are a made a bit easier as they still have a very low center of gravity. Therefore, toddlers will still utilize external assistance during most of their gait during this time. The toddler's gait is identified as a wide-based, short stepping walk with externally rotated features of the lower extremity. In an ironic move by mother nature, many older adults will adopt this same gait pattern when experiencing balance issues.

After about 4-5 months of upright walking, a more mature gait pattern with a more heel-to-toe hip extension will start to take form. This is the gait that will identify who we are for the rest of our lives.

It is interesting to note that each person's gait pattern is as unique as their fingerprint. So much so the Chinese government is heavily investing in artificial intelligence that will identify citizens by their gait rather than by facial recognition. To think that our most basic form of locomotion is inherently tied to who we are is just one of the many reasons that I find human gait endlessly fascinating.

Golden Gait Rule

It is commonplace for patients to report that they have previously been coached to walk a certain way by another medical practitioner. Perhaps they were told they need to place their foot a little more straight, push off their big toe, or a plethora of other neurotic cues. Outside of major neurologic insults such as stroke, trauma, or some other neurodegenerative disorder, gait coaching is akin to trying to change your personality.

Rather than creating false cues, a better approach to make functional, long-term change is to pay homage to Aristotle's quote, "the whole is greater than the sum of its parts". Thus, by working on joint mobility, central stability, or general strengthening, a practitioner stands a much greater chance of making a change to the 'whole.'

From a chicken or egg perspective, the jury is still out on whether bipedalism preceded the development of human intelligence or vice versa. Either way, we are forever joined with our innate locomotor drive, or at least we have been up until the past few decades.

Homo sapiens walked on average 6-10 kilometers per day for hundreds of thousands of years to forage, hunt, travel, and socialize. However, due to environmental and societal changes, we have lost touch with our foot-powered means of transportation, which may have more negative downstream effects than one might think. Since the advent of wearables and the 'quantified life,' it has become popular (to the extent of physicians prescribing this metric) to ensure you get 10,000 steps a day. From an anthropological standpoint this step count can be calculated by multiplying the average number of steps in a kilometer by approximately 8 kilometers (average of the historical 6-10 kilometers per day). The reality of the 10,000 step count comes from a Japanese watchmaker. Who drove the popularity of this number for purposes of marketing his brand, yet again we must follow the money.

Marketing and FitBits aside, walking a moderate amount each day is essential to optimized human health. Evidence reported in the Journal of the American Medical Association (JAMA) showed that 4400 steps per day were the minimum steps needed to deliver positive health benefits. Any more steps than this showed only a nominal benefit, but it is worth noting that it did not show any harmful effects either.

So what are the magical benefits of going out for a walk? For starters, that same study out of JAMA, which had over 18,000 women participants, showed a 40% decrease in premature death. Not too shabby. Walking is also correlated with improved cardiovascular health, staving off dementia and Alzheimer's, and improving social bonds. Once again, movement is programmed into our DNA, and to deny our nature can ultimately lead to the decline of our health and possibly even our eventual demise.

I digress, back to the toddlers.

Utilizing efficient central stabilization strategies the toddler can now start to wind up the fascia, or connective tissue, that ties all of the muscles, tendons, ligaments, bones, and even organs all together. This is the true magic of human movement, allowing for our meager strength and wobbly upright posture to produce elastic energy return necessary for walking, running, and throwing.

Toddlers tap into this efficient energy return by producing more cross body or contralateral patterning when walking, where the opposite side arm and leg swing in unison. They can also begin negotiating stairs, although at this age they will usually step one foot to each stair at a time. As gait becomes more consistent, the hands become even freer to continue to explore the environment. For this reason, around 18 months of age, hand preference will start to emerge. Whether your baby is destined to be a southpaw or a righty, they will typically begin to throw objects with both hands before the age of two.

Thus at this stage, we now have our modern-day hunter-gatherer. A toddler can walk upright, navigate multitudes of terrain, interact with their tribe, chuck implements at would-be prey, or maybe just a Lego at the unsuspecting forehead.

If we had to give this developmental phase a name other than 'toddler,' it may suffice to term it the 'imitation' phase. Imitation plays a crucial role in beginning the process of learning the necessary skills to maintain survival. In modern times we may not face the same struggles or environmental rigors as our hunter-gatherer predecessors. However, the ability to imitate is still crucial for the demonstration of social integration and higher-level cortical function.

In order to mimic parents, siblings, and others at this age, humans have developed a unique network of neurons called the mirror neuron system. As the name implies, it is theorized that mirror neurons are an ancient evolutionary adaptation that allowed us to become one of the world's greatest imitators and actors. According to research from the Journal of Natural Science, Biology and Medicine, 2012, the mirror neuron system primarily develops before 12 months. Therefore, it is vital to mimicking various movements and behaviors.

It is theorized that mimicking others also allows a young one to develop empathy and understanding of others. According to biologist and naturalist E.O. Wilson, this empathetic imitation is part of the process of 'sociobiology'. Contrary to a model that bases human behavior solely off of the interplay between mind and culture, sociobiology theorizes that our internal biology is one of, if not the greatest, drivers to the development of behavior throughout life. Regardless of the what theory we use to prop up the development of social behavior, the process is still ubiquitous throughout most of the human population.

The complexity of human communication is intriguing, and when we look at how we actually get our message across we circle right back to the vital importance of movement. Joe Navarro is a former FBI counterintelligence officer and expert on nonverbal behavior and author of the book *What Every Body is Saying*. Navarro, and many other experts in the field, believe that upwards of 90% of human communication is nonverbal. "Having conducted thousands of interviews for the FBI, I learned to concentrate on the suspect's feet and legs first, moving upward in my observation until I read the face last," Navarro notes of his investigative process.

While mimicry is vital to proper development, it can also open up opportunities for unwanted imitation. All parents have faced the embarrassment of a child repeating a not-so-appropriate word or catching a derogatory gesture that seemed to go unnoticed at the time. Beyond these somewhat laughable incidents, children at this young age are like cortical sponges. Therefore, the way we move, interact, talk, breathe, and play all significantly impact a toddler for years to come. Just as John Connolly states in *The Book of Lost Things*, "for in every adult there dwells the child that was, and in every child there lies the adult that will be".

Mimicry can also present as isopraxism, or the almost impulsive synchrony of action observed in humans as a way of showing preference, indifference, and even disgust with others. There is an interesting phenomenon that translates isopraxism into the realm of walking gait, called synchronized walking. Research shows that walking synchrony can take as little as five minutes to occur, and it is far more common when physical contact, such as holding hands, is part of the equation. As with most things that have evolutionary sticking power, walking synchrony provided utility in the days of hunting and gathering. Large game, water, or other heavy loads would need to be shared between others, and when the tribal duties of daily survival are shared, social bonds strengthen and once again the whole becomes greater than the parts.

As cliché as long walks on the beach with a loved one might seem, this encapsulates what walking is to humans–a mode of travel, a social bonding experience, a genetic link to our to the millenia old library of human movement. Walking is the movement that makes us human, and I think Helen Keller said it best, "Walking with a friend in the dark is better than walking alone in the light".

5
2-3 Years

"Where the speech is corrupted, the mind is also."
- Sencea

Now that a child can walk the walk, it's time to talk the talk. Communication can be distilled down to movement in its simplest form, whether it's sounding out a word with our mouth, writing a letter or phrase, or even signing a symbol. These movements are crucial to interact and thrive in human culture. Around the second year of life, most toddlers can use sentences containing 2-3 words. So, even though they could speak before this age, this is the first time we see fully expressed unique thought delivered in a somewhat comprehensive manner. In other words, we can now not only use movement to express the context of our inner workings, but we can now vocalize the exact thoughts we are having.

We do not often think of human speech as a movement, but it may be one of the most complex human movements ever devised. With coordinated movements from our tongue, lips, and vocal cords, we produce sounds and then form those sounds into shapes to create reproducible and representative communication we call speech.

The Language of Newborns

Do you ever have a thought that stops you dead in your tracks? Such as, "what language do newborns think in?". Yeah, a real mind-bender. It is theorized that newborns utilize logic, reason, and pattern recognition to build cognitive processes that contextualize their surroundings and existence. However, some researchers believe that this primitive idea-based thinking has to be 'dumbed down' with the adoption of human language, as the ability to express complex ideas and patterns is not conducive to verbal or written language.

Recall from our earlier stage of 0-6 months that the importance of tummy time was centered around proper development of the shoulder girdle and creating synergistic relationships with the surrounding anatomy. Spending time in a prone position is also crucial for the process of speech development, more precisely, the breathing patterns necessary for speech.

When a baby progresses through the phases of uprighting, higher levels of coordination must be achieved between the thoracic diaphragm, pressurization within the abdominal cavity, spinal stability, and ultimately extremity movement and control. A significant differentiator of humans from many other mammals is the ability to uncouple breathing from movement. It is this uncoupling that also allows us to create sounds and words. If we could not uncouple our breathing from movement, we would always sound like someone trying to speak into the microphone after just finishing a marathon, not ideal, to say the least.

In addition to breath control, their is a symphony of movement coordination that takes place to utter a single word. The formation of ideas into speech takes place in Broca's area within the left hemisphere of the brain. Then the arcuate fasciculus and cerebellum help synchronize the movements of jaw, tongue, and lips to form words and speak clearly. Each sound and word that passes over our lips, and often take for granted, is a literal masterpiece of human movement.

The Hidden Epidemic

In the 1930's Weston A. Price, a dentist at the time and now a legacy figure in the nutrition field, was busy traveling to tribal villages around the globe to examine their dental health. During his time in Polynesia, Alaska, and Africa, Price began to theorize that populations reliant on mainly processed foods, the Western diet, were more likely to have tooth decay, malformed dental arches, and changes within the soft palate. Price's thinking was directed at the nutritional differences within the diet, but further research has elucidated a more mechanical means of dysfunction.

In their book *Jaws: The Story of a Hidden Epidemic*, Sandra Kahn and Paul R. Erlich, a pioneering orthodontist and a world-renowned evolutionist, respectively, further explore the increasing prevalence of micrognathia (small lower jaw), high-arched palates, and increased lower facial height. This presentation has been termed "long-face syndrome" and is strongly associated with mouth breathing, obstructive sleep apnea, and bevy of other maladies.

Price was the first to beg the chicken or egg question when it came to these changes. Does the way we breathe and what we eat determine structure, or vice versa? While issues such as cleft palate or other genetic disturbance in face and jaw structure surely change breathing and eating patterns, for the general population it is usually our jaw mechanics and breathing that lead to structural changes.

Processed food is just that, processed, it takes a large amount of mastication or chewing process out of eating. Our ancient hominid cousin, *Paranthropus boisei*, nicknamed "Nutcracker Man" had large jaws and a ridge on top of its skull where the masseter, the strongest muscle in the body, attached. Evidence of the tough fodder it subsisted on such as roots and raw nuts. When children survive on a diet of pureed everything and hyper-palatable processed food, they become devoid of the stressors necessary to challenge the muscles of mastication which in turn help develop the jaw and palate.

But it's not just dietary changes that lead to our shrunken-heads, the way in which we breathe may be an even more important contributor to our facial structure. In his aptly title 1882 book *Shut Your Mouth and Save Your Life*, George Catlin wrote, "When I have seen a poor Indian woman in the wilderness, lowering her infant from the breast, and pressing its lips together as it falls asleep...I have said to myself, 'Glorious education! Such a mother deserves to be the nurse of Emperors". This is in stark contrast to many babies and even adults today who remain unaware of their mouth based respiration. By not utilizing nasal breathing we create a scenario

that is ripe for facial structure changes and long-term breathing dysfunction.

Along with voluntary control of speech, it is around this time that most toddlers also gain better awareness and control of their ability to urinate and defecate, or at least every parent hopes. Voluntary control of the urinary system and bowels may not be thought of as a part of the course of movement development, but all of the movement pieces of the puzzle needed to be put in place before conscious continence could occur.

With over 40 different sphincters and four major diaphragms, humans are a giant tube that constantly equalizes fluid and air pressure to dictate the desired outcomes. Common dysfunctions within these sphincters and diaphragms can present as urinary incontinence, acid reflux, and even sleep apnea.

The ability to ambulate allows a baby to move out of their mess, but also, a great deal of pelvic floor control must be obtained before altogether ditching the diapers. Using the bathroom on their own is just one more piece of creating movement independence, and as most parents will attest, it is a very welcome independence day.

If you have ever happened upon a two or three-year-old playing with a dog, there is a good chance that you'll find a barking, four-legged version of a child with a very confused canine looking on. Imagination is now splashed onto the canvas of mimicry like a Jackson Pollock painting. This interplay between fantasy and reality is vital to movement development as toddlers copy playmates, parents, and animals. This process also allows toddlers to explore themselves and their environment in different conceptual context. And it gives me a fair bit of relief, seeing as I thought I was a dog for a few years early on in life, see mom, totally normal!

Independence and exploration within a child's environment allow for more fine motor development as toys and instruments become more intriguing. I don't know how many of us can remember learning to tie our shoes, but it can be quite a frustrating process for the uninitiated. Temper tantrums are quite common at this age, hence the label of the 'terrible twos'. Emotional development during this time is in hyperdrive as a child learns how to cope within more complex social constructs beyond their family.

If you have ever dreamed of your child going to the Olympics, this is the stage to start the training. Please do not 'train' your child to do anything. All joking aside though, the youth sports environment is quickly becoming more professionalized, and numerous studies show that early specialization leads to more injuries and poorer overall athleticism. So, would it not be better to just to let kids be kids? And what do kids like to do? You guessed it, triathlon. Okay, maybe not, but by the age of three, most children can proficiently swim, ride a bicycle, and run.

Humans have deep ties to the water. Proponents of the 'Aquatic Ape Hypothesis' go so far as to theorize that our divergence from our great ape ancestors was due in part to our relationship with the water. As humans fostered a deep bond with the water, we began to develop a multitude of aquatic adaptations. For example, simply placing your face in cold water stimulates the mammalian dive reflex which helps shunt blood to our core and lower our heart rate in order to prioritize reduced oxygen consumption for prolonged breath holding. While our breath holding capabilities pale in comparison to many of our sea-dwelling mammal cousins, a 56-year-old diver recently set a new world record breath-hold at 24 minutes and 33 seconds!

Infants (0-5 months old) possess two other unique reflexes that show our ancient connection to water. The diving reflex allows infants to hold their breath when placed underwater automatically. Also, when placed stomach down in the water, the swimming reflex allows arm and leg movement that mimics swimming. Both of these reflexes will start to fade around the 6-month mark, and after this time, swimming and breath-holding need some guidance to achieve proficiency.

When explaining the ease of doing something, we sometimes use the idiom "it's like riding a bike". Riding a bike may be part of the aforementioned intergenerational transference because it does seem as if almost everyone knows how to and seldom ever forgets. Cycling can become so hard-wired into our movement DNA that it can become a therapeutic agent. For example, Parkinson's patients that suffer from 'freezing gait' or the inability to walk often still retain the ability to ride a bicycle with ease and grace. The reciprocal and fluid motion of biking is thought to tap into rhythmic patterns within the damaged part of brain called the basal ganglia.

While riding a bike requires a machine to achieve maximum efficiency, perhaps the greatest form of human locomotion will finally emerge around three years of age. Humans' ability to run is such a unique movement when compared with the rest of the animal kingdom. So much so that to fully understand running, we must take an anthropological trip back in time.

6
3-5 Years

"The real purpose of running isn't to win a race,
it's to test the limits of the human heart."
- Bill Bowerman

When looking at the fossil record, it seems as if Homo erectus literally ran right out of the hominid family tree, and jogged all the way toward modern-day humans. One of our early evolutionary ancestors, Aurstralopithecines, shows evidence of bipedal walking around 4.4 million years ago. Still, it was not until a full 2 million years later that bipedal running made an appearance. While modern-day great apes can sprint for very short distances on two legs, endurance running for humans requires an entirely different set of traits and anatomical adaptations.

Even though humans have been utilizing all of these evolutionary gifts to run for over 2 million years, researchers still cannot fully agree on *why* we started to run in the first place. One of the leading theories as to why genus Homo adopted running is that it may have been helpful for competitive scavenging or persistence hunting. This theory is rooted in the idea that humans had to use teamwork and endurance to steal food from other mammals or run down large prey over long periods of time without fangs, claws, or any other natural weaponry. This led to humans evolving bigger, more elastic tissues, the ability to sweat, a variety of energy systems to cycle through, and improved upright stabilization. Eventually leading to Homo sapiens becoming the most dominant endurance mammals the world has ever seen.

When diving deeper into the anatomy that allows us to run, we find that the ability to wind up and release energy through major tendons such as the Achilles decreases energy output during running by up to 50%, versus using pure muscular contraction to push and pull us along. Other tissues such as ligaments and fascia also play a vital role in efficient energy return. At approximately four years of age, children will have a fully formed medial longitudinal arch of the foot. The medial arch utilizes the ligaments and tendons of the foot to create a spring-like effect with both walking and running.

Shoes

Shoes are a seemingly endless void of discussion when it comes to the topic of running. So, let us take a quick journey into the void. Modern-day shoes, running or leisure, are rarely designed for how a human foot has evolved, instead they tend prioritize aesthetics rather than improve function. Shoes create a scenario where our feet are forced to adapt to ill-fitting containers, which can lead to bunions, atrophied muscles, and many other dysfunctions and injuries.

Shoes can also act as 'deprivation chambers,' where the limitations placed on the foot create decreased feedback through the almost 7000 free nerve endings in each foot. Numerous studies show that shoes, particularly stiff-soled children's' shoes, can change natural gait patterns. For children under the age of three

choosing shoes with no sole such as moccasins is ideal. Once children engage with things like asphalt and other unnatural surfaces that require a bit more protection, it is best to find shoes with a wide toe box and flexible soles that allow for adequate foot movement within the shoe.

Shoes may be necessary for the majority of our life, but spending time outside shoes is crucial for proper function and improved health. For example, a study out of the University of Hamburg showed that going barefoot leads to improved motor development, not just through childhood, but possibly for the decades to come.

As for choosing a running shoe in adulthood, it simply comes down to comfort. In a literature review looking at all shoe-fitting data for the past 20 years, Benno Nigg, Ph.D., determined that shoes do little to improve performance or reduce injuries. The best advice for finding the optimal shoe was to choose one that was comfortable. An additional study out of Australia found that upwards of 50% of people were in too-small of a shoe; most importantly, shoes were usually found to be too narrow rather than too short. So do your children and yourself a favor and stay out of shoes as much as possible, and when shoes are warranted, find shoes that are comfortable and fit appropriately.

As strange as it may seem, our ability to cool ourselves down by sweating may be one of the more vital adaptations humans ever encountered when it comes to our endurance capabilities. Over a few hundred thousand years Homo erectus and eventually Homo sapiens started to shed body hair and in its place develop an elaborate system of eccrine or sweat glands. Our ability to sweat and replace that lost sweat with water and electrolytes, in essence, creates one of the best liquid-cooled radiators the world has ever known. This cooling process takes advantage of a physics principle known as the heat of vaporization, whereas most other mammals have to pant or use surface-level vasculature to cool themselves down.

Our proclivity for either sprint or endurance-based activity is primarily determined by genetics, early life activities, and specific training throughout a lifetime. While genetic and muscle fiber-type testing to determine this penchant does exist for children and adults, the data is still inconclusive as to how accurate, or pertinent this testing is for implementing specific training. Nevertheless, humans' energetic flexibility is a marvel of nature, allowing us (the most elite) to sprint in excess of 28 miles per hour or even run 100 miles in as little as 14 hours!

To establish this wide range humans have evolved to utilize glucose and glycogen to produce intense bouts of strength and power or switch over to fat and even protein utilization when faced with extremely long bouts of endurance. Much of the energy processing in our bodies occur within the 'powerhouse' of our cells, the mitochondria. Research shows that mitochondrial health is imperative to overall health and longevity. Mitochondrial dysfunction is now thought to be one of the major players in neurodegenerative diseases like Alzheimer's and dementia. It is possible to increase the number of mitochondria present in the body, and this is best done through bouts of long endurance but at relatively easy effort levels.

The earlier that children partake in endurance-based activities, the bigger and better the aerobic engine they build. Which has a plethora of health benefits throughout life, beyond making them endurance aficionados. So am I saying to start training your child for a marathon? Absolutely not. Once again nature trumps nurture with the appropriate answer. Play.

You would be hard-pressed to find a 4-year-old doing a 30-minute cardio session on a treadmill, let alone any other animal taking part in needless bouts of endurance. With little to no coaxing, though, you will see a young child play for hours on end, mixing in running, jumping, crawling, climbing, and various other movements, all of which help develop a variety of systems in addition to aerobic capacity.

Children rarely play by themselves if they have the option. One of the keystones of these developmental periods is the simultaneous glimpses of independence and specific social networking beyond the family. Around the age of five, children will start to form specific friends rather than interacting with any child within their vicinity.

Social bonds outside of the family have actually been determined to be one of the essential factors in longevity and happiness, especially later in life. The foundation of friendship is genuinely formed during these early years, and much of that social behavior is rooted in movement and play. So perhaps we should learn from our younger generation and keep moving, playing, and doing so within a tight-knit group of friends. That maybe one of the best prescriptions for optimal health.

Even though humans' relationship with running has existed for hundreds of thousands of years, that relationship has become strained in just the last century or two. In the U.S., about 15% of adults identify running as one of their main activities of choice. Of that 15% or 50 million people, over 80% will experience some type of running-related injury annually. So a pre-programmed evolutionary movement connected to both play and fun as a child, has now become a painful burden. This disconnect is primarily driven by environmental factors such as early and prolonged exposure to sitting, lack of physical education in school systems, and increased sedentarism.

Whether it was a group hunt or participating in a foot race with your tribe, running as with walking, has always been a social behavior. As our relationship with running has deteriorated so do the social bonds that drew us to run together. People are now wound up in metrics, miles, and social media likes when it comes to the their running endeavors. While this is not all bad, it is further evidence that as the environment around humans continues to shift, it will continue to alter our relationship with our evolutionary past. So it begs the question, as we evolve away from our intimate social connections and endurance excellence, are we in fact becoming less human. If so, could running toward the wisdom of our ancestors be the answer?

7
5-8 Years

"Give me a child until he is 7 and I will show you the man."
- Aristotle

To think that in the first 2,555 days of life, the foundation of your child's personality, character, and movement vocabulary is primarily determined for the remainder of their life. Without hard science to back his proclamation, Aristotle was not far off the mark. By the age of 5, 90% of the brain's capacities are formed, and it will not be until approximately two decades later that the frontal cortex will fully develop. We hone and develop our cognitive and movement abilities for a lifetime, but much of how we perceive and interact with the world will be determined relatively early in life.

With most of the hard wiring in place by the age of 5, the period between 5 to 8 years old is a time of immense cognitive development. Most of the knowledge and experience acquired and processed during this time is done so while children are in a brainwave state called theta. Theta brain waves are present in almost everyone when dreaming, sleeping, praying, or meditating, but children under the age of 8 spend most of their waking life in this brain wave pattern. Theta brain waves are thought to be correlated with imagination, creativity, emotions, and intuition. Hypnosis subjects also display these same brain wave patterns.

This hyper-suggestible period is vital; children use their imagination and creativity to develop their beliefs and the framework of their perceived worldview. This time is also essential to the development of a child's subconscious mind, and it is thought that the subconscious processes at ten times the rate of our conscious mind and regulates as much as 95% of our waking life. Subconscious processing allows us to operate within our modern-day environment optimally, which tends to inundate us with thousands of daily inputs and outputs. The subconscious allows us remain largely unaware of how we are reacting to each stimulus within our surroundings. Still, this cognitive adaptation frees up our executive function to make critical decisions and maintain space for creative output.

Children are unknowingly patterning everything in their cortex, dependent on what interactions and environmental settings present themselves. Research has shown that children will mimic everything from parental gestures, laughs, and walking gait. At least once per week in my clinic, a patient tells me their bunions are "genetic". I hate to burst the genetic bunion bubble, but this is not quite the case. While genetic attributes such as tissue laxity, foot arch morphology, and the prevalence of inflammatory arthritides can all set the stage for functional and structural change at the big toe, there is no specific bunion gene. Far more common drivers of these changes are footwear and possibly learned paternal or maternal walking and running gait patterns.

I do not want any parent to feel they are guilty of bunion transference abuse, as this is not a matter of genetic or epigenetic expression. Instead, bunions are a perfect example of subconscious movement mirrors that extend into the realms of posture, preferred exercise, and even pain patterns, and these have much more to do with environmental reflection than genes. Research from the *American Psychologist* showed that chronic pain complaints tended to cluster in families where a mother or father was affected by headaches or low back pain. This concept is known as an ecological model of chronic pain, where the chances of pain are drastically increased when raised with a parent dealing with pain or other health issues. Further exacerbation of the ecological model occurs when parents catastrophize pain they experience or their child encounters.

There is obviously room for debate on whether this is purely an environment-based outcome or not. A lifestyle lacking the promotion of healthy eating or exercise can ultimately lead to poorer health outcomes. Nurture or nature always lands at the center of topics such as this. But in the case of movement development, it simply becomes a case of being aware of how you are nurturing your nature. Your child is consciously and subconsciously watching for hints of success or failure on your journey to survive within the environment. It would behoove us all to use this knowledge as a catalyst to extend our movement vocabulary and prioritize our health. After all, it is for the greater good of all humanity, no pressure though.

Hypermobility

Hypermobility, or the ability to move joints beyond their normal range of motion, is thought to affect 10-15% of children under the age of 10. While this percentage continues to climb, the question of actual prevalence versus examination effect needs to be posed. Are there in fact more hypermobile children today than there were a decade ago, or is the medical world better acquainted with this

concept and therefore "finding more" hypermobile children through normal examination.

I think there is a bit of both scenarios at play, but if there is truly an increase in extra bendy kids, the real question is why? For starters, if you do not stress the musculoskeletal system you will develop a body that lacks the resiliency needed to handle the daily rigors of life. It is almost akin to an astronaut returning from a zero gravity environment. The lack of stress on the astronauts body prompts a quick response via their physiology to preserve calories and energy by decreasing muscle mass and bone density.

So if a child is raised in an environment where sitting on the couch for six to eight hours a day, the U.S. equivalent of zero gravity, then we must realize that the expected outcome would be a softer, more bendy, and less movement adept organism. Beyond the lack of movement nutrition, other factors such as environmental endocrine disruptors both in utero and throughout early life can definitely play a role in collagen formation and repair.

Hypermobility goes beyond just being more flexible though. A 2020 study out of BMC Musculoskeletal Disorders explains that the prevalence of hypermobility was three times higher in children with anxiety disorders. Not only does this become a musculoskeletal health concern, but now we are looking at a systemic issue. Should we really be surprised though? After all we are simply a system of systems, and on the path to holistic health we know that we must tend to body, mind and soul.

So get your kids moving and get moving with your kids.

This stage of development has also been coined the "stage of industry" by developmental psychologist Erik Erikson. During these years, children readily learn new skills, focusing on the process rather than the end result. This process-driven state is something that Robert Greene discusses in his seminal book *Mastery*. Greene states that "Masters return to this childlike state, their works displaying degrees of spontaneity and access to the unconscious, but at a much higher level than the child".

Without refined motor skills, it makes sense that the end product is of less importance than the process. It is the process of repetitive gross and fine motor movements with intense bouts of focus that refine and hone our movement patterns. This phase tends to be when children can get lost in play with toys or others for long periods. These intense bouts of play often take precedent over eating, drinking, or sleeping. Interestingly, within self-help circles, it is standard advice to harken back to these childhood playtimes and ask this question in order to help unearth your true purpose or calling in life. What did I become so immersed in as a child to the point of skipping meals to do so?

So, it could be surmised that this is a purpose-building period. We are establishing our self-identity both at a conscious and subconscious level and determining where exactly we fit into social and environmental constructs. Just as our world seems to be coming into a bit of focus, nature starts to turn the physiological knobs and dials.

8

8-12 Years

"That's the real trouble with the world, too many people grow up."
- Walt Disney

Being a child that grew up in the nineties, I believe that I witnessed the greatest era of professional basketball there has ever been. Legends such as Shaquille O'Neal, Patrick Ewing, and Michael Jordan graced the hardwood during a time when basketball reigned king. While all of those hall of famers were over 6-foot-5, a 7-foot-1 player from Key West, FL, holds the record for the biggest growth spurt of any NBA player. David Robinson, AKA' The Admiral', played for the San Antonio Spurs and was a league MVP, multiple-time All-star team member, and two-time NBA champion. In a single year, David grew an astonishing 10 inches between his junior and senior years of high school! Then Robinson grew another 6 inches while playing for Navy, topping him out at his imposing 7-foot-1 frame. This type of growth spurt is abnormal, but the incredible ability of the human body to accelerate growth before, during, and after puberty can be both a blessing and a curse.

There are three fundamental phases to childhood growth:
• A rapid decelerating infantile growth phase lasting until approximately age 3.
• A prolonged childhood phase with a steady height increase.
• The adolescent growth spurt can be followed by some latent growth up to the approximate age of 25.

There are wide variances of exactly when children hit these phases, and for this reason, it is critical to pay heed to both chronological age and developmental age. Chronological age is a child's actual age, while developmental age is the aggregation of physical, mental, and emotional maturity. Thus, a child with a chronological age of 12 years may possess a biological age of anywhere from 9 to 15-years-old! My wife may say that my chronological and developmental age gap is even greater than that.

The difference between a 9-year-old and a 15-year-old is enormous. Therefore it is imperative to monitor growth correctly, and yes, it goes beyond just marking height on the door frame. The Canadian Sport for Life program has created a system for doing just that with their youth athletes. By tracking data points such as standing and sitting height, arm span, and weight, the Canadian group can better determine when growth spurts are occurring–allowing them to dictate how exercise and training should be programmed based on such.

In the U.S., we have seen a 5-fold increase in youth sports injuries since just 2000. One would think that all of the advancements in sports medicine and an overall decline in youth sports participation would result in far fewer injuries. However, the famed orthopedic surgeon Dr. James Andrews has been educating the public on why he believes so many injuries are occurring in youth athletes. Andrews was quoted as saying, "it comes down to two main factors: specialization and professionalism". The club model for youth sports has popularized the notion of early specialization and paired that with year-round 'developmental' leagues.

If we go back to the early nineties once again, it was common for children to play multiple sports, each having its defined season and subsequent offseason. You may have the occasional all-star or traveling team that extended a season by a few weeks, but all-in-all, children were expected not to be specialists and also to take breaks. To have time to simply be kids. Dr. Andrews noted that it is a pretty simple solution to get ahead of the problem, "Give them time to recover, please, give them time to recover".

Benjamin Franklin has been credited with the axiom of "an ounce of prevention is worth a pound of cure". This gets to the heart of programs like the Canadian Sport for Life growth tracking system. Adding the curveball of growth spurts into the milieux of year-round play, with only slight variance in sport or movements, is a perfect recipe for pain and injury. Unfortunately, the current model of youth sports is probably here to stay, so the best option in most parents' and physicians' eyes is to do our best to protect children within the existing youth sports environment.

By determining what phase of growth a child is in, it is possible to plan the best times to take breaks from sport and allow for the natural accommodation of movement. Detailed tracking programs have the added benefit of letting parents and coaches know exactly what type of movement or skills to work on and when. During each phase of growth, specific attributes are primed to either be honed or possibly lost forever.

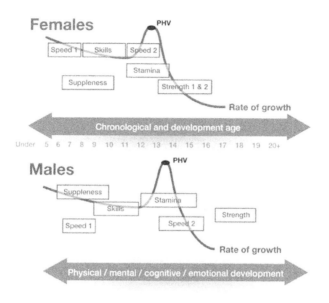

Figure 5. Windows of Accelerated Adaptation to Training (Balyi and Way, 2005)

The five 'S's of training; speed, skill, suppleness, stamina, and strength, give us a lens through which to view the training and development of youth through growth spurts. The trainability of speed, skill, and suppleness (flexibility) is primarily determined by chronologic age. All three attributes are to be maintained and developed before the onset of Peak Height Velocity (PHV) or the top of the growth spurt curve. While this time period includes working on things like sprinting, jumping, hitting, and throwing, all of these are operating on the foundation of functional and full-range of motion. If the range of motion or flexibility is hampered in this phase due to too much specific training or play, it can be challenging to regain in later years.

The fourth 'S', stamina, becomes of critical importance at the beginning of PHV. It is not uncommon knowledge within the strength and conditioning world that a big aerobic engine helps out in almost every other aspect of training. During PHV, we have seen many of the most dominant endurance athletes, such as Lance Armstrong (seven consecutive Tour de France victories, albeit some possible PED assistance), Kate Courtney (first American in 17 years to win the overall UCI MTB World Cup Title), and Michael Phelps (28 total Olympic medals), hit their stride with aerobic capacity. It is intriguing to point out that ancient cultures have understood the importance or prioritizing aerobic work at young age for thousands of years. The ancient Greeks called this "fatigue work", and this made up the bulk of daily work or training for youth until around the age of 20. Building a big aerobic engine is also vital to help develop the last 'S', strength, during this period.

Within the early specialization of youth athletes and club play programs, it has become increasingly popular to work on strength training as an adjunct to practice and play. While that is a great idea in theory, we have shown why it needs to be implemented appropriately and with the proper foundation previously laid. Modern-day children, on average, have weaker grip strength, are less flexible, and have worse aerobic conditioning than their parents did at their age. This scenario sets the stage for an even more unstable environment to introduce generalized strength training aimed at improving performance. Rather than the intended outcome of strength and conditioning programs being improved performance and decreased injury we actually tend to see the exact opposite occur.

The concept of injury prevention is a hotly debated within the medical and sports performance fields. With a polarized division of those who think we should be working towards that goal, while others think it is virtually impossible. While I do agree that injuries, in particular in sport, are inevitable. What should not be an expected outcome during childhood is pain and movement dysfunction without trauma or other justifiable causes. The framework laid out for the management of youth movement during growth spurts needs refining, but we still have to start somewhere.

While the best laid plans for honing the five 'S's' can help stave off unnecessary injuries, it is still normal to feel disconnected from our bodies during these rapid developmental periods. Like a baby giraffe just getting their legs under them, movement this time is uncoordinated and spastic. We may not remember it, but we all went through that 'awkward' movement phase. It does get better, but before we make our way out of the tumultuous jungle of our teen years, nature has one more hormonal trick up her sleeve that will make the awkwardness of our preteen growth spurts seem relatively insignificant.

Here comes puberty.

9
12-18 Years

"What war has always been is a puberty ceremony."
- Kurt Vonnegut

Rites of passage occur at four typical periods throughout a human's life: birth, puberty, marriage, and death. Each passage signifies us leaving one version of ourselves behind to ascend to the next stage of life, or in essence, a 'movement' to higher versions of ourselves. Sadly, in Western culture, we are largely deprived of rites of passage for the pubertal transition. Yet, this is arguably the most vital transition as it begins to shape our position and role in society and life in general as a man or woman.

The classic Jewish Bar and Bat Mitzvahs, the Vanuatu land divers, Amish Rumspringa, and my favorite, the Native American vision quest are just a few examples of the many different types of adulthood transition rites of passage ceremonies across history and culture. These ceremonies are vital to the individual and demonstrate to the tribe or community that the individual has made this critical leap into adulthood.

Coined by 19th-century anthropologists, the term "vision quest" describes a spiritual journey, often referred to among Indigenous nations as "dream visions" or "dream fasts". Participants, often adolescents, are said to receive sacred knowledge and strength from the spirit world. Practiced as a rite of passage among some Indigenous cultures in North America, such as the Blackfoot, Cree, and Inuit, vision quests reflect the role of spirituality and contemplative thinking in Indigenous cultures and provides an essential connection between the participant, the Creator, and nature. This ritual process usually occurs around the age of 12 to 13, which typically coincides with the onset of puberty for both males and females.

Quite a stark contrast from modern-day Western culture, where a set of braces, acne-riddled skin, and an increased sexual drive are mere signals that are socially recognized and, therefore, a semblance of transition is assumed. Humans seek order, and in particular, creating order in terms of how they fit into the world. In a more chaotic and confusing world than ever, it may be worth reintroducing actual rites of passage back into the culture. After all, the term 'adulting,' meaning to do things that adults regularly have to do, did not appear in the everyday lexicon until 2009. A lack of recognizable transition has led to an entire generation of humans that feel lost as to their place in time and culture, which ultimately shapes the greater framework of society, for better or worse.

Take a Breath

Speaking to an entire generation that feels lost as to their place within society, walking hand-in-hand with that social ambiguity is often anxiety. According to the National Institutes of Health, nearly 1 in 3 of all adolescents ages 13 to 18 will experience an anxiety disorder. When you think about it, the increased prevalence of anxiety almost seems logical.

Constant bombardment by social media, disparaging news cycles, increasingly competitive college entrance standards, it seems like the logical outcome of all of these increasingly negative inputs would find a teen living in a sympathetic, fight or flight, state. While some of the environmental and technological inundation could definitely be eschewed or monitored by parents and teachers. The actual root of the issue is that we are leaving children largely devoid of tactics to handle normal stressors of daily life, let alone the tidal wave of 21st century reality.

"I felt like I was trapped in a respiratory research spin cycle. Different scientists, different decades: the same conclusions, the same collective amnesia". This is James Nestor's explanation from his book *Breath,* for how he was baffled by the fact that every couple thousands of years the importance of breathing, along with age old breathing practices seems to resurface into the mainstream. When the topic of anxiety arises, a chicken or egg scenario is ultimately presented. Does anxiety precede breathing dysfunction or does breathing dysfunction precede anxiety?

Is it biology or psychology that rules the roost when it comes to determining our state of mind. It is definitely a question without a concrete answer at this point in time, but what we can ascertain is the interesting trend in three seemingly distinct areas of human health. We have already highlighted the increased prevalence of anxiety, but also on the rise by 39.8% since 1990 are breathing disorders. Along with both of these maladies we have seen a popular culture upswell in the interest of breathing performance.

Breathing gurus, classes, and books just like Nestor's have come about not just by chance, but by probable cause. Breathing and anxiety are intimately connected, and many would debate that breathing is upstream of anxiety most of the time. Seeing as how many of the non-medication treatment options for anxiety revolve around the regulation of the one autonomic nervous system action we can take voluntary control of...our breath.

There is a broad range for the onset of puberty; anywhere from 8-years-old to almost 15 is considered normal. Boys typically begin puberty a bit later than girls, but in today's environment, filled with growth hormone-laden food and endocrine disruptors, both sexes experience earlier and earlier onset. As a result, what used to be called 'precocious puberty' or early onset signs of hormone change are becoming more commonplace with children, and this often comes at a price. According to Frank M. Biro in the journal Pediatrics, girls that experience early-onset puberty are typically not as tall later in life, experience higher rates of depression, and are even at higher risks for certain types of cancer.

At this pivotal point in a human's life, movement essentially becomes aimed at attracting and eventually procreating with a mate. As primal as this may sound, the sexual drivers behind specific movements and body aesthetics will dominate a sizable portion of a human's life. At this age, each sex begins to become a subconscious sexual movement detective. For example, males start to both consciously and subconsciously warrant more attention to the manner in which a female's widening hips move as she walks or runs, as this may determine fertility. Whether or not she displays grace and balance as she runs through the park or plays basketball with friends, this can be evidence of body control that may be necessary to keep children safe. Even the way a girl brushes her hair away from her face affects how a boy perceives her interaction with him and other potential suitors.

For females, their attention is diverted to how a male walks. Does he walk with poise and confidence, which may signify virility? Do the way his broadening shoulders rotate as he walks display the ability to protect both her and their potential offspring? Even the subtleties of how other boys move around one another can reveal to girls a possible testosterone pecking order among the tribe.

Observing a group of teens interact during this time, it can sometimes be surprising that humans have made it this far. Boys, pumped full of testosterone and operating with a frontal cortex primed for poor decision making will often show-off or "peacock" for girls with acts that borderline on stupidity and often risk bodily harm. While girls, seemingly more reserved, are culturally persuaded to start participating in enhancing their appearance through a new focus on things like clothing and makeup. Both of which are actually utilized to enhance movement. Whether the goal is to draw attention to lips through added color or breasts through lower cut tops. The draw to the opposite sex comes from the way in which the body moves around these accentuated attributes.

As I mentioned, much of this movement analysis takes place in the subconscious, but for the hormone-fueled pubescent, it may seem like the opposite sex is all they can think about. This period is where things like dancing change from simply a way to express how one is feeling through motion to a way to display sexual competency in a manner that is deeply rooted in the human psyche. Every culture throughout history displays some evidence of various types of music-driven mating rituals. It may be a hard pill to swallow for parents out there, but that 7th-grade dance is the Western version of the African Wodaabe courtship dance. This may change your mind about volunteering to be a chaperone at the next Spring Fling.

Sweat-inducing hip gyrations synchronized to a bass line that keeps a couple in rhythm together; this is our first foray into partner pseudo-sex. Dancing is both a way to determine if a mate is suitable and at the same time 'practice' what it takes to procreate. If you are "lucky" enough to have seen the movie Napoleon Dynamite, you may recall his surprising and quirky high school talent show dance moves. His seductive, snowboot-wearing sways were enough to pique interest from 'Deb.' Allowing her to look past his evolutionary lack of prowess in many other categories. Dancing, particularly with the opposite sex, is one of the oldest ways to gauge the suitability of a partner. It is a skill that is the culmination of movement coordination and control. Mother nature is a funky mother indeed.

When not participating in the village rave, our hunter-gatherer ancestors were usually hard at work procuring food, building weapons, or traveling to find or follow roaming food. Yet, our modern Western society exists during a time where very little manual labor is required for survival. This type of work was typically what developed the bodies of adolescents, putting their hormone surges to good use–eventually developing both their bodies and their competency within society and the potential family unit. Nowadays, we are often forced to retreat to a fluorescent-lit gym, with bass-thumping music motivating us to sculpt our physiques and improve our physical fitness. These teen years are the first time we may see human movement being honed or altered by the drive to improve one's physique to impress the opposite sex.

While being aesthetically driven to exercise is not necessarily bad, gyms and machines have massively derailed human movement. Greece is the motherland of what we now know as the modern-day gym. The word 'gymnasium' originated from the Greek word "gymnos'" which translates to naked. That translation makes the yoga pants, and shirtless peacocking of modern gyms seem tame in comparison. Gyms at that time were usually a place for the education of young men (it will be a while until we get to women in the gym), which included physical education, scholarly pursuits, and bathing (yes, nude). In addition, the ancient Greeks designed these public gymnasiums for athletes to train for open games such as the Olympics.

Sculpting the body became looked at as narcissistic, if not downright sinful, during much of the Dark Ages. Then we see a bit of a resurgence of gymnasiums in 1800's Germany, but it was not until the early 1900s in the U.S. that we saw the rise of the proper gymnasium. The average man or woman frequented these early gymnasiums, but comparing what was done within those early gyms, with the practices of modern gyms could not have been more different.

It was not uncommon for a business person, perhaps a member of the New York Athletic Club, to stop off for an hour session of rope climbing, rings work, pommel horse, and a bit of boxing before heading back to the office. On a daily basis, members of these prescient gyms were doing what we currently reserve for elite gymnasts. The idea of fitness was led by function, or more accurately usefulness. People still recognized the need to maintain strength, speed, and stamina throughout their life, for the purpose of recreation, but more importantly for the times when a helping hand was needed.

Even 26th President, Teddy Roosevelt continued to box with soldiers, swim across the Potomac, and trek through rugged landscapes throughout his presidency and beyond. But, over the course of two world wars, a boom in industrialization, and commoditization of everything in the West, we saw a massive shift in how people moved and, therefore, the types of movement they practiced.

In the 1970's Arthur Jones finally culminated his search for the "thinking man's barbell" when he created the Nautilus fitness machine. Mr. Jones was a chain-smoking, overweight, business tycoon who was far more concerned with profit margins rather than improved physical fitness. The Nautilus machine set the stage for the detachment of natural human movement from exercise for the next few decades. This growing chasm has led to many issues within our modern society. There has been a bevy of exercise machines developed over the last 50 years, everything from the Bowflex to Suzzane Somer's Thighmaster, and it is not as if these machines are downright sinister or useless. Instead, they tend to compartmentalize human movement and aid movement inefficiency and dysfunction rather than promoting functional human movement.

In just the last decade, there have been massive shifts in what equipment and setting people exercise: the explosion of CrossFit, boutique fitness chains such as OrangTheory, endless variety of yoga options, and now in-home virtual exercise options like Peloton or Mirror. As humans, we inherently seek out a relationship with movement, no matter how novel or alien. Still, the industries that prop up the next fitness fad or a guaranteed six-pack apparatus, usually take us further from a genuine relationship with movement. This dysfunctional relationship begins in our earliest experiences with exercise, movement, and sport, but the echoes of this bond will follow us into adulthood and for decades to come.

10
18-40 Years

The Dalai Lama, when asked what surprised him most about humanity,
answered "Man! Because he sacrifices his health in order to make money.
Then sacrifices money to recuperate his health."

It could be a dilapidated house in a small Texas town or an obese mother of three trying to reclaim her health. In America, we are intoxicated with the idea of reimagining, remodeling, and redoing. I applaud the idea of salvaging and repurposing when it comes to homes and small towns, as this lies in stark contrast to much of our consumer lives, where we feel pressure to get the newest clothing, phone, and car every few years. When it comes to our health and movement, though, a fixer-upper mentality means that at some point along the way, we have lost something extremely valuable. We may actually lack the ability to renovate and restore our health and movement to its prior optimal function.

In my neck of the woods, I call this phenomenon the 'Iron Tribe Effect.' Iron Tribe is a very successful cousin to CrossFit that lends itself to small group and individual high-intensity interval training. Iron Tribe's pricing creates a clientele with unique socioeconomic factors, and in my opinion, a generally shared concept of health and fitness. Many of the individuals within our local gym are well-to-do business owners, executives, or professionals such as lawyers and physicians.

Professional Posture

Since your mother first scolded you for not sitting up straight, to the modern-day demonization of sitting, posture seems to be front and center when it comes to our movement journey. You have probably heard that, "sitting is the new smoking". After the release of a paper from the University of Leicester reported that adults who spent 50-75% of their day sitting had a significantly increased risk of diabetes, heart disease, and stroke. This became quite the click-bait-worthy headline, not to mention that correlating sitting to an almost 50% increase in all-cause mortality will scare you right out of your seat.

While posture has much more to do with how we move in general, the positions that we adopt regularly do impact our movement. From elementary school through college, children spend a large part of each day seated, we then sit at work for the next few decades, and in between all that sitting, we sit down to relax when we get home. When we spend this much time performing a task, we adapt, for better or worse. So whether it is stiffness in your hips, upper back, or ankles, how you move will ultimately dictate your posture. I think Robert Schleip, MD captures the idea when pontificating on the importance of fascia when it comes to posture. "Fascia is like the St. Bernard of the body, slow and loyal, responding slowly to responses over time".

The best way I have found to explain this is using the concept of absolute value. Yes, I am taking you back to 6th-grade math class. The absolute value of a number is its actual magnitude without regard to its sign. In terms of posture, think of it like this. If your upper back is supposed to be able to extend about 35 degrees (bending backward), and after years of accommodating to desk work and a seated posture your upper back can now only extend 25 degrees, your nervous system is now likely to set a new start point to keep the absolute value or magnitude of movement the same.

So how would you get that 10 degrees of movement back? Well, by increasing the forward flexion of your spine by that 10 degrees, so that now when you bend back, voila, you have your 35 degrees of 'perceived' upper back extension. While thinking about your posture is not a bad thing to be aware of, a much more helpful way to improve your posture, in the long run, is to ensure that you can move adequately in all planes of motion. Incorporating Pomodoro breaks, or breaks every 25 minutes or so, with some generalized movement throughout your work day can go a long way to warding off the plight of desk work. Add to that some strength training aimed at creating movement variability and you're well on your way.

The common thread among many of these gym-goers is that they sacrificed their health to gain ground within their profession. This trade-off allows them the financial and time freedom at this juncture in their lives to attempt to regain their health. The period from post-college to early thirties can be one of the most transformational times of any human's life. Marriage, children, and careers are all competing for our time and energy; people tend to 'let themselves go' to keep up with it all. As a result, lifelong habits surrounding diet, exercise, and overall health are formed during this period. Leveraging this habit-forming time to our advantage can reap benefits for the rest of our lives. Still, a lack of focus on health at this phase often results in obesity, acquired disease, and reduced quality of life.

According to the Bureau of Labor Statistics, as of 2019, less than 20% of the U.S. adult population exercises regularly. When combining the percentage of overweight and obese adults in America, the figure is approximately 74%. One could surmise from looking at this data, albeit without valid cross-referencing available, that the 20% of exercising adults lie outside of the overweight 74% of the rest of the country. Uri Ladabaum, MD of Stanford, sums it up nicely "we cannot draw conclusions about cause and effect from our study, our findings support the notion that exercise and physical activity are important determinants of the trends in obesity".

How do we stay on track during this period of intense change and demand? Much of what happens during this period of our life was set in motion almost a decade earlier. According to the team at Project Play in Aspen, CO, adolescents who play sports are eight times as likely to be active at age 24 as adolescents who do not play sports. While we cannot go back in time, we can lead by example and implement strategies with our children that help them form a positive relationship with movement and exercise for years to come. Some of the best ways to motivate adults to start an exercise regiment are no different from those that would entice children to play. It has been shown that adults that participate in intramural sports, group-based exercise, or even simply walking with a friend or family member are twice as likely to make exercise a long-term habit.

Did you get your steps today? This question did not enter our daily lives until the last decade. Technology contributes to our more sedentary life in many ways, but new developments in wearables and exercise tracking have proven beneficial for motivating people to exercise. Most of the metrics, that devices such as FitBits or Apple watches use, are centered around steps or simply the amount of movement that an individual performs. This can be great to aid in the initiation and habituation of exercise, but it leaves a giant piece of the health paradigm out. Movement.More precisely, the ability to move freely in all planes of motion without pain, becomes rarer and rarer as we age. Even though this may be common, it does not mean that this is normal.

As we age, we rarely realize what we are losing in terms of movement until it matters most. Pain or injury without traumatic insult is a familiar part of Western life, as highlighted in Part I of this book. The process that brings us to the 'straw that broke the camel's back' point, is a winding journey of sedentarism and lack of awareness. A sure-fire way to increase awareness of our movement is to move outside of typical exercise. Just as a child playing tag may run, jump, crawl, or climb to evade their pursuer, adults need to explore movement variety daily. Unfortunately, this ideology runs counter to the typical exercise regimes of most modern humans. Typically we hop on a treadmill, bike, or in a pool to move in one direction, most often the sagittal plane (forward and backward), and clock our 45 minutes of exercise. Even when lifting weights, most people exercise in the sagittal plane, and even then, we rarely see a full range of motion expressed throughout the movements.

While he played a major role in the disparaging shift in focus of exercising for physique rather than function, bodybuilder and Hollywood icon Arnold Schwarzenegger, was ahead of his time when he coached people to perform weighted exercises through a full range of motion to ensure joint and tissue mobility. As with most things in modern times, the pendulum always swings back the other way eventually. The machine-based gyms and exercise routines that dominated my childhood are now being challenged with the reintroduction of things like kettlebells, natural movement classes, and a plethora of stretching and mobility classes to ensure your leopard-like suppleness. These are definitely steps in the right direction but still lend themselves to contrived attempts at the human version of a fixer-upper. The best way to reach your golden years healthy and intact is to never lose your fitness or movement competency in the first place.

11
40-75 Years

"The man who has lived the longest is not he who has spent the greatest number of years, but he who has had the greatest sensibility of life."
- Jean-Baptiste Rousseau

"Those that are disabled from work by age and invalidity have a well-grounded claim to care from that state". This was a quote from German Chancellor Otto von Bismarck in 1889 when he first described the concept of retirement. His initial motivation was to aid in the employment of the abundance of unemployed youth at that time. Many countries, including the U.S., soon followed suit, giving rise to government-backed financial aid programs for those of a certain age.

For many, the word retirement is synonymous with a time in our life when we can finally enjoy the fruits of our labor. We expect to be less stressed, surrounded by family and friends, and able to pursue hobbies and interests that we may have put off during the few decades we traded our time for the prospect of future financial freedom. This period of life is now called the 'Third Age,' which is classically defined as a period between retirement and the beginning of age-imposed physical, emotional, and cognitive limitations. The concept of the Third Age is a relatively new period in human history as increased lifespan has created a new gap between middle-age and old-age.

I will admit that this age range is a bit peculiar. It seems that the differences between a 40-year-old and a 70-year-old can be immense. The truth is that we see a higher prevalence of acquired illnesses and musculoskeletal dysfunction at much earlier ages, which sadly closes this age gap. For the first time since 2006, we have seen a slight decline in life expectancy, and at the same time a precipitous decrease in health-span. Health-span being defined as how many years of our lifespan we live free from disease or disability. This rift is a major cause of concern, not just for those entering this period of life but for the healthcare policymakers and administrators who are now severely malpositioned to handle the impending tsunami of disability, dysfunction, and disease.

According to CDC data from 2009, by the time you reach the age of 55 in the U.S., you will have acquired at least two chronic health issues and be on at least four prescription medications. It is estimated that if the average American wants to retire by age 65, they would need at least $400,000 just to cover medical expenses for the remainder of their life. Those 'golden years' may be instead turning into 'gold-plated years'.

After the age of forty, one of the first significant health milestones that takes place is the massive shift in hormones in both men and women. Just turn the TV on for a bit, and you are inundated with commercials promising to increase testosterone, improve libido, beat back hot flashes, and help create what I call a 'second puberty.' As with almost any capitalist action, this is simply the market answering the need of the consumer.

Just as with precocious puberty, the onset of these normal hormonal changes in both sexes is happening at alarmingly earlier points in life. The average age of the onset of menopause is now 40, with perimenopausal symptoms often occurring in women's mid-thirties. Men even see symptomatically low levels of testosterone as early as age thirty!

Both of these hormonal shifts are normal, but the age at which they are now happening is not. As men age, it has been theorized that it is advantageous to decrease testosterone to soften our demeanor for improved interaction with children and grandchildren. This may be true, but when testosterone begins to decline too early in life, a plethora of health issues can surface. Such as obesity, brittle bones, and cholesterol dysregulation, not to mention the apparent effects that decreased sex hormones have on male libido, mood, and vigor for life.

Menopause is a normal cessation of menstrual cycles that signals an end to the ability to procreate. Easily identifiable by hot flashes, decreased libido, and the occasional irritability or anger. Again, a typical process within a human's lifetime can wreak havoc when initiated too early. Issues with decreased bone density, increased risk for breast and cervical cancer, and increased risk for all-cause mortality have all been associated with early-onset menopause.

Bone Density

A widespread health concern among the aging population is decreasing bone density. As a result, it is now standard practice for females over fifty to receive an annual DEXA (dual-energy X-ray absorptiometry) scan to ensure their T-score is within normal limits. This is also becoming a popular addition to men's yearly visits as we see a decline in bone density across sexes.

Is decreased bone density normal as we age? Yes, but not to the extent that we see in Western culture. A few factors result in our

societal brittle bones which can result in increased stress and acute bone fractures. Two leading causes of early and rapid osteoporosis are decreased mineral content or uptake from the diet and an overall decrease in skeletal stress or loading.

The dietary issue stems from a depleted mineral base within the soil and poor dietary choices throughout a lifetime. As for loading your skeletal system to obtain the desired outcome of increased bone density, that is where the U.S. lags far behind. In many Blue Zones worldwide, we see that a decreased incidence of osteoporosis is also linked to an increased amount of physical labor throughout a lifetime. So if you want to maintain strong bones, you have to supply your body with the correct micro and macronutrients, but you must also challenge your musculoskeletal system in order to get it to respond accordingly.

So, what is the game plan during this period of life to keep from becoming a health statistic? From a physical health standpoint, a sound strategy needs to be implemented in our forties to ensure that we maximize our health-span and lifespan into the Third Age. This strategy includes weekly bouts of aerobic exercise, resistance training, movement diversity, and social interaction.

The first step to improve your hormonal health is to ensure that resistance exercise is part of a weekly routine. Lifting moderate to heavy weights, better yet when combined with complex, multi-joint movements (squats, deadlifts, etc.) one or two days per week, has been shown to increase levels of anabolic hormones, specifically testosterone, growth hormone, and insulin-like growth factor-1 (IGF-1). These hormones are vital to offsetting the natural bone and muscle loss that occurs later in life. In addition, this hormone cascade also improves your body's sensitivity to catecholamines such as dopamine, epinephrine, and norepinephrine which have downstream effects on mood, cognition, pain regulation, and vascular health.

After the age of 30, the average man's maximum attainable heart rate declines by about one beat per minute per year, and his heart's peak capacity to pump blood drifts down by 5%-10% per decade. That's why the average healthy 25-year-old heart can pump 2½ quarts of blood a minute, but a 65-year-old heart can't get above 1½ quarts, and an 80-year-old heart can pump only about a quart, even if it's disease-free. In simple terms, this diminished aerobic capacity can produce fatigue and breathlessness with modest daily activities. For this reason, we must incorporate some form of aerobic exercise into our regiment upwards of three to four times a week.

Aerobic exercise creates resistance on the vascular walls and increases demand on the pulmonary system. This allows for improved vascular elasticity, enhanced vascular performance and sprouting of microvascularization throughout the body. As a result, aerobic exercise is a crucial component to reduce atherosclerosis, regeneration of tissues and bones, and improving aerobic efficiency at rest. In addition, aerobic exercise helps regulate LDL and HDL cholesterol relationships, creates a cascade of neurochemicals that can help with depression and anxiety, and has even been shown to decrease the likelihood of dementia and Alzheimers.

In the U.S., we have a bit of a disharmonious relationship with aerobic training. It is not uncommon to find people that despise steady-state cardio work, and on the other side of the coin, we find people who have taken a good thing too far. Using running as an example, we see that most people either run too much volume or run too hard for the distance they typically cover. If we use the standard 5-zone heart rate system, most people exercise within zone 3 or 4 almost 90% of the time. Many of the previously mentioned benefits of aerobic exercise are gleaned from spending around 80% of the time in zone 2 exercise. This zone is characterized by a conversational pace of running or even a brisk walk, typically ranging from 45 to 90 minutes in duration. A far cry from the hard-charging, breathless pace that most people think is necessary to improve endurance.

In a similar aspect to the one day a week of heavy resistance training, one day per week can be reserved for a more challenging and possibly shorter aerobic effort. This is where things like high-intensity interval training, moderate resistance training with less rest between sets, plyometrics, and even sprinting are great options. These forms of exercise are often centered around power, which is applying strength or force in short bouts of intensity. Interestingly, one of the first movements to escape our movement vocabulary as we age is the ability to jump. Which is a perfect example of human power, and thus the focus on the metric of vertical jump height in many different sporting arenas.

So far, we have filled five to six days of our week with quality movement, but even the best-laid plans can fall prey to a lack of variety. While building strength, endurance, and power, it is critical to create space for movement diversity. The variation we seek could simply come from switching up the resistance and aerobic exercises or settings in which they are performed each week, or it could come from a seasonal approach to exercise. Let your activities ebb and flow with the seasons. This marriage can have the added benefit of entwining your health endeavors with the outdoors, which can improve mood, sleep, and immune activity as we sync with the diurnal flow of each changing day.

We have an iron-clad plan for improved health and lifespan by taking our weekly strategy and sprinkling in the magic ingredient of social interaction. A study out of Tokyo Medical University which examined differences in elderly individuals who exercised alone versus those that exercised with others, showed that regardless of the amount of exercise, more benefits were seen from training in groups. Our goal in the 'golden years' of our life is to enjoy ourselves, free of disease and disability, all while setting ourselves up for a seamless 'jump' into that final phase of life.

12
75+ Years

"Our nature lies in movement; complete calm is death."
- Blaise Pascal

Jeanne Calment was 122 years and 164 days old when she finally passed away in 1997, making her the longest living person in modern human record. When examining Jeanne's amazing life, many people want to anecdotally attribute her longevity to her post-dinner Dunhill cigarette and small glass of port wine. What may have been more contributory to her ability to outlive both her children and grandchildren were her daily prayers, visits with friends, and various movements routines.

Jeanne awoke at 6:45 each morning and performed a bout of 'gymnastics.' These were not backflips or bar routines but instead a series of whole-body stretches. Nurses at the facility where she stayed for the last three decades of her life noted that she seemed to move "faster than residents 30 years younger than her". Jeanne also continued to ride her bike until the age of 100, which was only brought to an end by an ankle fracture. From which she recovered quickly and still maintained the ability to walk.

There are outliers in every facet of life, and it is quite possible that Jeanne Calment's routines, diet, and self-care played no significant role in her longevity. Instead, she may have been genetically gifted and downright lucky. But when looking at studies on Blue Zones, areas across the globe where people live the longest, we find that Jeanne abided by many of the central tenets of these longevity epicenters.

National Geographic fellow and explorer, Dan Buettner, and his team traveled the globe to study Blue Zones such as Sardinia, Italy, Okinawa, Japan, and Loma Linda, California. By exploring the cultural practices in these locations, they compiled a list of practices that led to more centenarians in these areas than anywhere else on earth. The list is as follows:

1. **Move naturally.** The world's longest-lived people do not necessarily exercise; instead, they live in environments that constantly nudge them into moving without thinking about it. They grow gardens and do not have mechanical conveniences for house and yard work.

2. **Purpose.** The Okinawans call it *Ikigai*, and the Nicoyans call it plan *de vida*; for both, it translates to "why I wake up in the morning."

3. **Downshift.** Even people in the Blue Zones experience stress. Stress leads to chronic inflammation, associated with every significant age-related disease. What the world's longest-lived people have that others do not are routines to shed that stress. Okinawans take a few moments each day to remember their ancestors; Adventists pray; Ikarians take a nap, and Sardinians do happy hour.

4. **80% Rule.** *Hara hachi bu*–the Okinawan 2500-year old Confucian mantra said before meals remind them to stop eating when their stomachs are 80% full. The 20% gap between not being hungry and feeling full could differ between losing weight or gaining it. People in the Blue Zones eat their smallest meal in the late afternoon or early evening, and then, they do not eat any more the rest of the day.

5. **Plant-based.** Beans, including fava, black, soy, and lentils, are the cornerstone of most centenarian diets. Meat–mostly pork–is eaten on average only five times per month. Serving sizes are 3 to 4 oz, about the size of a deck of cards.

6. **Alcohol.** People in all Blue Zones (except Adventists) drink alcohol moderately and regularly. Moderate drinkers outlive non-drinkers. The trick is to drink 1 to 2 glasses per day, with friends and/or with food. And no, you cannot save up all week and have 14 drinks on Saturday.

7. **Belonging.** All but 5 of the 263 centenarians interviewed belonged to some faith-based community. Denomination does not seem to matter. Research shows that attending faith-based services four times per month will add 4 to 14 years of life expectancy.

8. **Family first.** Successful centenarians in the Blue Zones put their families first. This means keeping aging parents and grandparents nearby or in the home (it lowers disease and mortality rates of children in the house, too.). They commit to a life partner (which can add up to 3 years of life expectancy) and

invest in their children with time and love. (They'll be more likely to care for aging parents when the time comes.)

9. **Right tribe.** The world's longest-lived people chose–or were born into–social circles that supported healthy behaviors; Okinawans created moais–groups of 5 friends committed to each other for life.

While following these tenets, by no means guarantees we will make it past the century mark; it is an excellent framework for living a healthy and purpose-filled life for many years. I did not determine the order of this list, but, interestingly, movement is at the top. Even more intriguing is that it is not exercising that seems to be a primary catalyst for catapulting us towards the century mark, but instead natural movement woven into daily activities.

In Westernized culture, our societal landscape is largely devoid of natural movement. This is determined both by our physical environment and the demands of everyday life. Humans no longer need to grow their own food, carry water from the river, or walk to get where they are going. We can live an entire life with almost every aspect of life shaped in such a way that we constantly erode our relationship with movement. With movement scarcity comes declining health and shorter lifespans. So for the first time in human history, we must now make the conscious decision to make movement an integral part of our daily life.

If the Blue Zone strategy is out of your comfort zone, Peter Attia, MD's concept of the 'Centenarian Olympics' may be a better fit. Dr. Attia is a physician that focuses on the applied science of longevity and wellness, and he encourages people to think about the things they would want to do when they reach the age of 100. His personal markers for movement success at this age include being able to get up off the floor on his own, pull himself out of a pool, pick up small children, and lift a 30-pound suitcase into an overhead bin.

This list may not fit your goals for when you reach the century mark; that is why you are encouraged to create your own version of the Centenarian Olympics. Once you have developed your list, the idea is to work backward to establish what milestones would be necessary for each decade in order to reach your goal. Creating this plan helps steer people clear of simply trying to be fit and instead allows them to aim at a specific target.

One fundamental goal for everyone looking to make it to the century mark is mitigating the risk of falls. As simple as this seems, according to the CDC, falls are the leading cause of injury-related death among adults age 65 and older. Fall death rates also increased by about 30% from 2009 to 2018. Once again, we see the plights of modern-day society dragging us, or rather tripping us, towards an early grave.

In 2012 a team of Brazilian researchers published their findings on the sitting-rising test (SRT) in the *Journal of Preventive Cardiology*. The researchers had over 2000 participants try to sit down and rise from the floor without using their hands, arms, or knees to assist the process. The researchers determined that individuals requiring more than one hand or knee to help them had a two-fold higher death rate over the 6.3 year follow-up period. While this test is not a stand-alone predictor of longevity, it is at least some measure of musculoskeletal competency as we age.

So how do we improve our SRT score and reduce our risk of falls as we age? A study from 2017 out of the Frontiers of Neuroscience found that a 10-week balance training program could be extrapolated to 10 years of juvenescence, or the power to regain youth . So not only does balance training accomplish the goal of improving vestibular and propioceptive function, in essence it makes us younger. It's not as if it is the fountain of youth, but balance is at the core of human movement.

We have explored movement from the time we were in our mother's womb all the way to our long, last sleep. There is by no means a "one size fits all" approach to human health and movement along this journey. I would like to think that what I have proposed throughout Part II of this book can act as a general framework for how humans came to move the way they do, how that relationship has become fractured, and provide a principally-based guide to help lead us through a movement-filled and healthy life.

Part III

The Anthropokrisis

1
Conclusion

The age of man, the Anthropocene. The epoch that for better or worse is marked by our time upon the Earth. A time when we have begun to see the dismantling of the natural world, of our world. Mass species extinction, rapid climate change, and what seems like a new daily catastrophe, with all indicators of causality or at least complicity usually pointing back toward man.

You have probably heard it said or felt the effect yourself; the older you get, the faster time seems to go. This same paradox may hold true for the Earth. A typical geological epoch lasts approximately 3 million years, so the proposed ushering in of the Anthropocene in place of the Holocene after only 11,500 years may make the Earth feel like a geriatric planet. While I do not think myself bold enough to propose an entirely new epoch is already upon us, I do think we could stop and reexamine the period in which we live.

As stated previously, the Anthropocene translates to "new man". While that is fitting, I think a better term for raising awareness and inspiring action may be *Anthropokrisis*. The Greek *krisis*, the etymological cousin to our modern-day crisis, is defined as a turning point in a disease. That is the change which indicates recovery or death.

Recovery or death.

The distinction between the two could be left up to fate or come down to a decision. A decision simply means taking fate into your own hands, but once you have tugged on the rope of destiny, you better have a plan.

What is the plan?

Just as a river flowing over a a boulder in its path must divert around the stone. Neither path around the rock is right or wrong, just simply a path. I think we are seeing the same type of split occurring among the human race, or at least the split is coming. A figurative line in the sand between *Kins* sand *non-Kins*. The *Kins* or kinesthetics, are those people that are still aware of, and seek movement.

We are already seeing camps form around the ideas of artificial intelligence, digital consciousness, and the possibility of leaving our bodies behind for a bold, new, fully digital world. Our meat suits donned useless as the stream of one's and zero's converges with the very molecules of our DNA. A world that seems to be an evolutionary step forward for some, a complete fantasy to others, and somewhere in between reality exists. Technology is changing our world at a speed that is almost incomprehensible, and the rate of change does not allow us to assess the possible collateral damage of the benefits rendered by this change.

Humans have always relied on tools to improve efficiency in order to maximize their likelihood of survival. The tables are turning, as our tools seem to be creating a possible future where the greatest machine ever gifted to us could become obsolete. The *non-Kins* lean on the same information at hand to come to their conclusions about the direction that they think the world is headed. Changing climate, growing populations, a possible kill-shot from a meteor, all of which, seem like ample evidence to support the need to upload and eject.

Slowly but surely we are seeing another camp form. More precisely we are seeing a camp return. The flicker of campfire from within the camp of *Kins* has almost been completely snuffed out, but possibly just in the nick of time the flames are being fanned by the need to reconnect with what is most natural and vital to our survival.

Regenerative agriculture, living off the grid, trading automobiles for bicycles, and simply becoming more aware of breath, are all different versions of the movement towards human movement. By reacquainting ourselves with the primal sparks that illuminated a path towards the evolution of Homo sapiens we may be able to regain what has been lost. Reclaiming our title as the greatest species the Earth has ever known.

Kins will uphold the position that we have lost much of the wisdom that brought us to this inflection point. The lightning rod to that knowledge is our body. The greatest machine ever conceived. No rival. No match. We can upgrade, reboot and reinstall just as the best tech in the world can, we just have to remember how.

Home Sapiens, the greatest species to inhabit the Earth. That title should come with a hefty responsibility.

Humanity has been scarred numerous times by traumas such as war, destruction, and disease throughout the last few centuries. Our most recent calamity came in the form of SARS-CoV-2 or COVID-19. With much data on both the death toll and the efforts behind treatment and prevention being clouded by biased and politicized media reporting, it is hard to precisely determine the exact impact this virus has had and will continue to have on humanity. However, what we can definitively extract from our current scenario is how intimately connected humans are to the environment in which we live.

During the lockdowns at the height of the COVID pandemic, the planet as a whole experienced what a team of researchers deemed the 'anthropause' or the Great Pause. During this Great Pause, we witnessed a plethora of environmental shifts that cast a ray of bright light onto the dark shadow of the pandemic. Improved air quality, animals repopulating urban areas, and abandoned migratory routes being reestablished were just a few of the miraculous examples of nature's resiliency during this otherwise ominous time. This glimpse of ecological robustness can also be extrapolated to the current health dilemmas we face as a species. Thus, giving us a hopeful outlook for the journey that lay ahead.

The anthropause is technically defined as "a period of unusually reduced human mobility". So, the reduction of human movement somehow led to expedient global health improvement? While at the same time I keep arguing that reducing human movement is the most significant contributor to our own declining health. Well, that seems to completely contradict the entirety of this book up to this point, I'll admit, it seems like quite an oxymoronic scenario.

When zooming in on the situation at hand, we see that it was, in fact, the type of movement reduction, automobile, plane, and boat travel, that was the catalyst for this shift. While we were sitting at home on the couch binging the Marvel Universe in chronological order, just saying some people did that, not me personally. We paused, and the Earth finally got the chance to take a breath. A moment to renew herself in light of the damage done. But as soon as lockdown started to ease and mandates were lifted, we were right back to business as usual. Back to driving to work rather than riding a bike or sharing a ride. Ditching our daily home exercise session as the time demands of normal life were once again imposed. Back to the disconnect between our internal and external environments.

Charles Kettering, the famed inventor and head of research for General Motors, once said, "A well stated problem is half solved". So what is it exactly that we are dealing with? A team of researchers released a commission report in The Lancet in 2019 that examined the interconnected epidemics of obesity, undernutrition, and climate change. The team deemed this a synergistic epidemic or the "The Great Global Syndemic", and noted that this is "the paramount health challenge for humans, the environment, and our planet in the 21st century".

If Kettering's notion is true, and we are indeed living during the Anthropokris, then by definition we are at a self-imposed inflection point. A point in time where the impact we have had on the global environment could be the next great health crisis we deal with as a species. The authors of an editorial that appeared in journals including the New England Journal of Medicine and The Lancet warn that "health is already being harmed by global temperature increases and the destruction of the natural world." In addition, a paper out of Nature Medicine goes so far as to specifically implicate the increasing global temperatures to the increase of zoonotic spillovers such as COVID-19. In a statement regarding this editorial, World Health Organization chief Tedros Adhanom Ghebreyesus said, "the risks posed by climate change could dwarf those of any single disease".

Did we miss our window during the Great Pause? Our opportunity to reflect on how we could change our daily habits to have a positive outcome on our health and the health of our environment. I call this ruminative process 'Environmental Reflection.' The process of examining how your daily actions have a ripple effect throughout your internal, external, and global environments. Thereby helping us to better recognize that our health is a mirror of the health of our environment. This is no easy task, but in the current predicament that we find ourselves, I think some of the best advice may come from actor and self-proclaimed minister of culture Matthew McConaughey. McConaughey states "that the more the selfish we become, the more selfless we actually become... what's good for me is good for we." If his message rings true, then for change to occur for the greater good, it must become personal.

To lasso the ethereal and bring it into our own personal world requires action fueled by knowledge, we must first understand what our motivation for change is. In Simon Sinek's *Start With Why*, he breaks down WHAT, HOW, and WHY to better understand our reasons for doing what we do. Sinek explains that *what* we do is primarily regulated by the neocortex or the part of our brain responsible for rational and analytical thought. Hopefully, through reading the previous chapters of this book, you now understand *what* to do when it comes to movement throughout all ages for both you and your loved ones. Unfortunately, the *why* is a personal question and sometimes much harder to answer.

Basing your decision to change on topics discussed in this book or any other information or idea that inspires you to do so is excellent. I'm biased of course. However, this process may not have the staying power needed to weather the storm. We need to find intrinsic motivation to create the type of forward progress that is needed to move us closer to our desired goal. So instead, let our current decisions be dictated by knowledge and need, and allow our future decisions to be guided by optimized biology.

I genuinely believe that the evidence currently at hand, shows us that seeking the selfish goal of improving human health is at the center of remedying many of the world's most significant issues. By refocusing our lens on the goal of healthy individuals operating within a healthy environment, we can tip the scales toward multiple solutions derived from a few simple changes. Whether it is the obesity epidemic, mental health disorders, or environmental strain, the true lynchpin may be human health. And what lies at the center of human health?

Movement.

Humans have spent the last few centuries creating an utterly foreign environment compared to the previous hundreds of thousands of years. We have called this progress. No one will deny the technological, scientific, and economic advancement that has taken place throughout human history. But we should be careful to not confuse progress with adaptation. Adaptation, or evolution, does not assume that we are becoming better just because we grow more accustomed to our environment. The issues we face daily and that have been examined in this book are evidence of this fact.

The father of modern science, Isaac Newton, may have said it best "nature is pleased with simplicity". Can it really be that simple? A return to moving as nature intended? I believe so, and I hope this book acts as a simple but empowering guide to do just that. The truth of the matter is that knowledge is only as powerful as the action it inspires, and while the human movement began millions of years ago, the choice to take part in the age of movement is upon us now.

The Story Continues

There were many catalysts that led to me finally writing this book. Most came in the form of questions from patients. Repeating theme and gaps in knowledge about things that I thought should be commonplace throughout society. Although, as the early mornings of writing began to accumulate, I realized that I was actually writing this book as guide for my younger self. The 9-year-old boy who was told he would likely never run again. Who would never be like the 'other kids', let alone return to the same person I was prior to breaking my leg.

Through fate, happen-chance or pure dumb luck, an early spark was lit inside of me. A spark that lit a fire, allowing me to not only overcome all preconceived notions as it relates to my movement journey, but to completely surpass some of my wildest dreams. Not only do I run today, I have competed in well over one hundred races, and in many of those I have podiumed or won. This is not meant to be braggadocios, instead I look at what I've done as an example to my patients, my friends, and my family. An example of being your own health advocate, educating yourself about your body, and in the end believing that anything is possible.

Far more important than running, is the opportunity afforded to me to play a part in the health and movement journey of my patients. At a time when the health of our species, as well as the health of our planet, are both in dire straits, I can't think of a more profound way to impact someone's life than to guide them on a path to optimal health. I am acutely aware that there are a multitude of people out there, that find themselves in the same scenario that I once did. Regardless of age, sex, or the challenge they be facing, my hope is that this book may provide a glimmer of light along the way.

Beyond my own journey, and that of the people I help on a professional level, I find myself thinking more and more about the world that awaits my daughter. Her generation is predicted to be the unhealthiest population of humans the world has encountered.

What if their dismal destiny can change?

What if we all became just a bit better each day? Thereby, transforming ourselves and the world we live in. Creating examples of what is possible by fostering healthy lifestyles, abundant relationships, and a richer life overall. Is this all blind optimism in the face of a grim forecast? Only time will tell, but regardless of the long-term outcome, moving towards a better future starts with one small step in the right direction. So let's get going.

Citations

1. Daniel Lieberman, PhD. The Story of the Human Body: Evolution, Health, and Disease. 2013. Pantheon Books: New York

2. Richard Shine, Gregory P. Brown, Benjamin L. Phillips. *An evolutionary process that assembles phenotypes through space rather than through time.* Proceedings of the National Academy of Sciences Mar 2011, 201018989; DOI: 10.1073/pnas.1018989108

3. Phillips, B.L., Perkins, T.A. *Spatial sorting as the spatial analogue of natural selection.* Theor Ecol 12, 155-163 (2019). https://doi.org/10.1007/s12080-019-0412-9

4. Vargas, Constanza et al. Costs and consequences of chronic pain due to musculoskeletal disorders from a health system perspective in Chile. Pain reports vol. 3,5 e656. 10 Sep. 2018, doi:10.1097/PR9.0000000000000656

5. By Rabah Kamal, Giorlando Ramirez, and Cynthia Cox. How does health spending in the U.S. compare to other countries? KFF. Chart Collections Health Spending. Posted: December 23, 2020

6. Lay San Too, Matthew J. Spittal, Lyndal Bugeja, Lennart Reifels, Peter Butterworth, Jane Pirkis. *The association between mental disorders and suicide: A systematic review and meta-analysis of record linkage studies.* Journal of Affective Disorders, Volume 259, 2019, Pages 302-313, ISSN 0165-0327, https://doi.org/10.1016/j.jad.2019.08.054.

7. Kandola, A.A., Osborn, D.P.J., Stubbs, B. et al. Individual and combined associations between cardiorespiratory fitness and grip strength with common mental disorders: a prospective cohort study in the UK Biobank. BMC Med 18, 303 (2020). https://doi.org/10.1186/s12916-020-01782-9

8. Foster-Schubert, Karen E et al. Effect of diet and exercise, alone or combined, on weight and body composition in overweight-to-obese postmenopausal women. Obesity (Silver Spring, Md.) vol. 20,8 (2012): 1628-38. doi:10.1038/oby.2011.76

9. Booth, Frank W et al. Exercise and gene expression: physiological regulation of the human genome through physical activity. The Journal of physiology vol. 543,Pt 2 (2002): 399-411. doi:10.1113/jphysiol.2002.019265

10. Julianne Holt-Lunstad,Timothy B. Smith, J. Bradley Layton. Social Relationships and Mortality Risk: A Meta-analytic Review. July 27, 2010. https://doi.org/10.1371/journal.pmed.1000316

11. Marshall, Michael. *Timeline: The evolution of life*. New Scientist. https://www.newscientist.com/article/dn17453-timeline-the-evolution-of-life/

12. May LE, Glaros A, Yeh HW, Clapp. Aerobic exercise during pregnancy influences fetal cardiac autonomic control of heart rate and heart rate variability. Early Hum Dev. JF 3rd, Gustafson KM. 2010;86(4):213-217. DOI:10.1016/j.earlhumdev.2010.03.002

13. Mette Juhl, MPH, Ph.D., Jørn Olsen, PhD Per Kragh, Andersen, dr.med.sci, Ellen Aagaard Nøhr, Ph.D., Anne-Marie Nybo Andersen, Ph.D. *Physical exercise during pregnancy and fetal growth measures: a study within the Danish National Birth Cohort*. Published: October 05, 2009.

14. Letsinger AC, Granados JZ, Little SE, Lightfoot JT (2019) Alleles associated with physical activity levels are estimated to be older than anatomically modern humans. PLOS ONE 14(4): e0216155.

15. Edward R Newton1 and Linda May 2. *Adaptation of Maternal-Fetal Physiology to Exercise in Pregnancy: The Basis of Guidelines for Physical Activity in Pregnancy.*1Division of Maternal-Fetal Medicine, Department of Obstetrics & Gynecology, Brody School of Medicine and Vidant Medical Center, East Carolina University, Greenville, NC, USA. 2 Foundational Sciences and Research, East Carolina University, Greenville, NC, USA.

16. Gema Sanabria-Martínez,1,2 Raquel Poyatos-León,1,2 Blanca Notario-Pacheco,2 Celia Álvarez-Bueno, 2,3 Iván Cavero-Redondo,2,3 Vicente Martinez-Vizcaino 2,4. Effects of physical exercise during pregnancy on mothers' and neonates' health: a protocol for an umbrella review of systematic reviews and meta-analysis of randomized controlled trials.

17. Roger L. Hammer, Ph.D. Jan Perkins, MSc Richard Parr, EdD, FACSM. *Exercise During the Childbearing Year.*

18. Valentina Chiavaroli, Sarah A. Hopkins, José G. B. Derraik, Janene B. Biggs, Raquel O. Rodrigues, Christine H. Brennan, Sumudu N. Seneviratne, Chelsea Higgins, James C. Baldi, Lesley M. E. McCowan, Wayne S. Cutfield, Paul L. Hofman. *Exercise in pregnancy: 1-year and 7-year follow-ups of mothers and offspring after a randomized controlled trial.*

19. Camilla Schou Andersen,1 Mette Juhl,2 Michael Gamborg,1 Thorkild I. A. Sørensen,1 and Ellen Aagaard Nohr3. *Maternal Recreational Exercise during Pregnancy in relation to Children's BMI at 7 Years of Age.* 1 Institute of Preventive Medicine, Copenhagen University Hospital, Øster Søgade 18,1, 1357 Copenhagen K, Denmark 2 Department of Public Health, Copenhagen University, 1014 Copenhagen, Denmark, 3 Section of Epidemiology, Institute of Public Health, University of Aarhus, 8000 Aarhus C, Denmark 7 October 2011; Revised 20 January 2012; Accepted 26 January 2012.

20. Linda E. May, Richard R. Suminski, Michelle D. Langaker, Hung-Wen Yeh, and Kathleen M. Gustafson. *Regular Maternal Exercise Dose and Fetal Heart Outcome.*

21. Elise L LeMoyne, Daniel Curnier, Samuel St-Jacques, and Dave Ellemberg. The effects of exercise during pregnancy on the newborn's brain: study protocol for a randomized controlled trial.

22. Beetham, K.S., Giles, C., Noetel, M. et al. The effects of vigorous intensity exercise in the third trimester of pregnancy: a systematic review and meta-analysis. BMC Pregnancy Childbirth 19, 281 (2019). https://doi.org/10.1186/s12884-019-2441-1

23. Lipton Ph.D., Bruce. Lessons from the Petri Dish. The Biology of Belief: Unleashing the Power of Consciousness, Matter, & Miracles. Hay House, Inc., 2016, p. 19.

24. Simon LV, Hashmi MF, Bragg BN. APGAR Score. [Updated 2020 Jan 25]. In: StatPearls [Internet]. Treasure Island (FL): StatPearls Publishing; 2020 Jan-. Available from: https://www.ncbi.nlm.nih.gov/books/NBK470569/

25. Peesay, Morarji. *Cord around the neck syndrome.* BMC Pregnancy and Childbirth vol. 12,Suppl 1 A6. 28 Aug. 2012, doi:10.1186/1471-2393-12-S1-A6

26. Gieysztor, Ewa Z et al. Persistence of primitive reflexes and associated motor problems in healthy preschool children. Archives of medical science : AMS vol. 14,1 (2018): 167-173. doi:10.5114/aoms.2016.60503

27. Daniel Wolpert: The real reason for brains - TED Talks, https://www.ted.com/talks/daniel_wolpert_the_real_reason_for_brains?language=en

28. The Mother and Child Health and Education Trust, http://breastcrawl.org/science.shtml

29. Javadi Parvaneh, V., Modaress, S., Zahed, G. *et al.* Prevalence of generalized joint hypermobility in children with anxiety disorders. *BMC Musculoskelet Disord* 21, 337 (2020). https://doi.org/10.1186/s12891-020-03377-0

30. Health Reports, Vol. 17, No. 3, August 2006 Statistics Canada, Catalogue 82-003.

31. Safe Kids USA Campaign. https://www.safekids.org/. 2009.

32. Centers for Disease Control. Healthy Schools Physical Activity Facts. https://www.cdc.gov/healthyschools/physicalactivity/facts.htm

33. JS Powell, KD Barber Foss, 1999. Injury patterns in selected high school sports: a review of the 1995-1997 seasons. J Athl Train. 34: 277-84.

34. Abderrazak El Albani, M. Gabriela Mangano, Luis A. Buatois, Stefan Bengtson, Armelle Riboulleau, Andrey Bekker, Kurt Konhauser, Timothy Lyons, Claire Rollion-Bard, Olabode Bankole, Stellina Gwenaelle Lekele Baghekema, Alain Meunier, Alain Trentesaux, Arnaud Mazurier, Jeremie Aubineau, Claude Laforest, Claude Fontaine, Philippe Recourt, Ernest Chi Fru, Roberto Macchiarelli, Jean Yves Reynaud, François Gauthier-Lafaye, Donald E. Canfield. *Organism motility in an oxygenated shallow-marine environment 2.1 billion years ago.* Proceedings of the National Academy of Sciences Feb 2019, 116 (9) 3431-3436; DOI: 10.1073/pnas.1815721116

35. Blatt G.J., Oblak A.L., Schmahmann J.D. (2013) Cerebellar Connections with Limbic *Circuits: Anatomy and Functional Implications.* In: Manto M., Schmahmann J.D., Rossi F., Gruol D.L., Koibuchi N. (eds) Handbook of the Cerebellum and Cerebellar Disorders. Springer, Dordrecht. https://doi.org/10.1007/978-94-007-1333-8_22

36. Francis Berenbaum, Ian Wallace, Daniel Lieberman, David Felson. *Modern-day environmental factors in the pathogenesis of osteoarthritis.* Nature Reviews Rheumatology, Nature Publishing Group, 2018, 14 (11), pp.674-681. ff10.1038/ s41584-018-0073-xff. Ffhal-01950118f

37. Varma, V. R., Chuang, Y. F., Harris, G. C., Tan, E. J., & Carlson, M. C. (2015). Low-intensity daily walking activity is associated with hippocampal volume in older adults. Hippocampus, 25(5), 605-615. https://doi.org/10.1002/hipo.22397

38. Wojtys E. M. (2015). *Keep on Walking. Sports Health.* 7(4), 297-298. https://doi.org/ 10.1177/1941738115590392

39. Acharya S, Shukla S. Mirror neurons: Enigma of the metaphysical modular brain. J Nat Sci Biol Med. 2012;3(2):118-124.

40. Zivotofsky, A. Z., & Hausdorff, J. M. (2007). The sensory feedback mechanisms enabling couples to walk synchronously: an initial investigation. Journal of neuroengineering and rehabilitation. 4, 28. https://doi.org/10.1186/1743-0003-4-28

41. Bramble DM, Lieberman DE. *Endurance running and the evolution of Homo.* Nature. 2004 Nov 18;432(7015):345-52. doi: 10.1038/nature03052. PMID: 15549097.

42. Wegener, C., Hunt, A. E., Vanwanseele, B., Burns, J., & Smith, R. M. (2011). Effect of children's shoes on gait: a systematic review and meta-analysis. Journal of foot and ankle research, 4, 3. https://doi.org/10.1186/1757-1146-4-3

43. Cranage, S., Perraton, L., Bowles, KA. et al. The impact of shoe flexibility on gait, pressure and muscle activity of young children. A systematic review. J Foot Ankle Res 12, 55 (2019). https://doi.org/10.1186/s13047-019-0365-7

44. Hollander, K., de Villiers, J. E., Sehner, S., Wegscheider, K., Braumann, K. M., Venter, R., & Zech, A. (2017). *Growing-up (habitually) barefoot influences the development of foot and arch morphology in children and adolescents*. Scientific reports, 7(1), 8079. https://doi.org/10.1038/s41598-017-07868-4

45. Buldt, A. K., & Menz, H. B. (2018). Incorrectly fitted footwear, foot pain and foot disorders: a systematic search and narrative review of the literature. Journal of foot and ankle research, 11, https://doi.org/10.1186/s13047-018-0284-z

46. Fattinger, S., Kurth, S., Ringli, M., Jenni, O. G., & Huber, R. (2017). Theta waves in children's waking electroencephalogram resemble local aspects of sleep during wakefulness. Scientific reports, 7(1), 11187. https://doi.org/10.1038/s41598-017-11577-3

47. Piqué-Vidal C, Solé MT, Antich J. *Hallux valgus inheritance: pedigree research in 350 patients with bunion deformity.* J Foot Ankle Surg. 2007 May-Jun;46(3):149-54. doi: 10.1053/j.jfas.2006.10.011. PMID: 17466240.

48. Palermo, T. M., Valrie, C. R., & Karlson, C. W. (2014). Family and parent influences on pediatric chronic pain: a developmental perspective. The American psychologist, 69(2), 142-152. https://doi.org/10.1037/a0035216

49. Sanders, J.O., Qiu, X., Lu, X. et al. The Uniform Pattern of Growth and Skeletal Maturation during the Human Adolescent Growth Spurt. Sci Rep 7, 16705 (2017). https://doi.org/10.1038/s41598-017-16996-w

50. Beaudoin C, Callary B, Trudeau F. Coaches' Adoption and Implementation of Sport Canada's Long-Term Athlete Development Model. SAGE Open. July 2015. doi:10.1177/2158244015595269

51. Peter A. Lee, Normal ages of pubertal events among American males and females, Journal of Adolescent Health Care, Volume 1, Issue 1,1980,Pages 26-29, ISSN 0197-0070, https://doi.org/10.1016/S0197-0070(80)80005-2.

52. Frank M. Biro, Louise C. Greenspan, Maida P. Galvez, Susan M. Pinney, Susan Teitelbaum, Gayle C. Windham, Julianna Deardorff, Robert L. Herrick, Paul A. Succop, Robert A. Hiatt, Lawrence H. Kushi, Mary S. Wolff. Onset of Breast Development in a Longitudinal Cohort, Pediatrics Dec 2013, 132 (6) 1019-1027; DOI: 10.1542/peds.2012-3773

53. Vallance, J. K., Gardiner, P. A., Lynch, B. M., D'Silva, A., Boyle, T., Taylor, L. M., Johnson, S. T., Buman, M. P., & Owen, N. (2018). Evaluating the Evidence on Sitting, Smoking, and Health: Is Sitting Really the New Smoking?. American journal of public health, 108(11), 1478-1482. https://doi.org/10.2105/AJPH.2018.304649

54. United States Bone and Joint Initiative: The Burden of Musculoskeletal Diseases in the United States (BMUS), Third Edition, 2014. Rosemont, IL. Available at http://www.boneandjointburden.org.

55. Barnes, S.F. (2011). Third Age - The Golden Years of Adulthood.

56. Kraemer WJ, Ratamess NA. Hormonal responses and adaptations to resistance exercise and training. Sports Med. 2005;35(4):339-61. doi: 10.2165/00007256-200535040-00004. PMID: 15831061.

57. Cardio exercise and strength training affect hormones differently https://www.sciencedaily.com/releases/2018/08/180824101138.htm

58. Morris, J. K., Vidoni, E. D., Johnson, D. K., Van Sciver, A., Mahnken, J. D., Honea, R. A., Wilkins, H. M., Brooks, W. M., Billinger, S. A., Swerdlow, R. H., & Burns, J. M.

(2017). Aerobic exercise for Alzheimer's disease: A randomized controlled pilot trial. PloS one, 12(2), e0170547. https://doi.org/10.1371/journal.pone.0170547

59. Gladwell, V. F., Brown, D. K., Wood, C., Sandercock, G. R., & Barton, J. L. (2013). The great outdoors: how a green exercise environment can benefit all. Extreme physiology & medicine, 2(1), 3. https://doi.org/10.1186/2046-7648-2-3

60. Buettner, D., & Skemp, S. (2016). Blue Zones: Lessons From the World's Longest Lived. American journal of lifestyle medicine, 10(5), 318-321. https://doi.org/10.1177/1559827616637066

59. de Brito, L. B. B., Ricardo, D. R., de Araújo, D. S. M. S., Ramos, P. S., Myers, J., & de Araújo, C. G. S. (2014). Ability to sit and rise from the floor as a predictor of all-cause mortality. European Journal of Preventive Cardiology, 21(7), 892-898. https://doi.org/10.1177/2047487312471759

61. Sandra V. Kahn and Paul R. Ehrlich. Jaws!: The Story of a Hidden Epidemic. Publisher: Stanford University Press, Hardcover £ 19.99, pages: 190. ISBN: 9781503604131

About The Author

Beau Beard DC, MS

A chiropractor, educator, and explorer, combining all of these passions into one focus of exploring the edges of human potential. TEDx speaker, author of 'The Age of Movement', and co-founder of The FARM, Beau is continually learning and educating with the aim to improve upon and even change the central concepts surrounding human and environmental health.

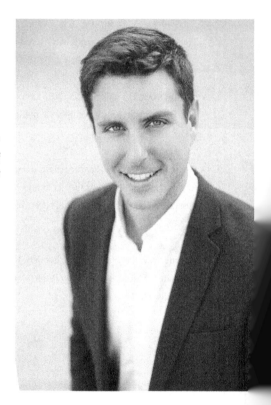

Made in the USA
Monee, IL
21 November 2021

82481480R00075